CELIA C. HISEY

Wellness Beyond 40

Intermittent Fasting for Men and Women – Your 21-Day Plan

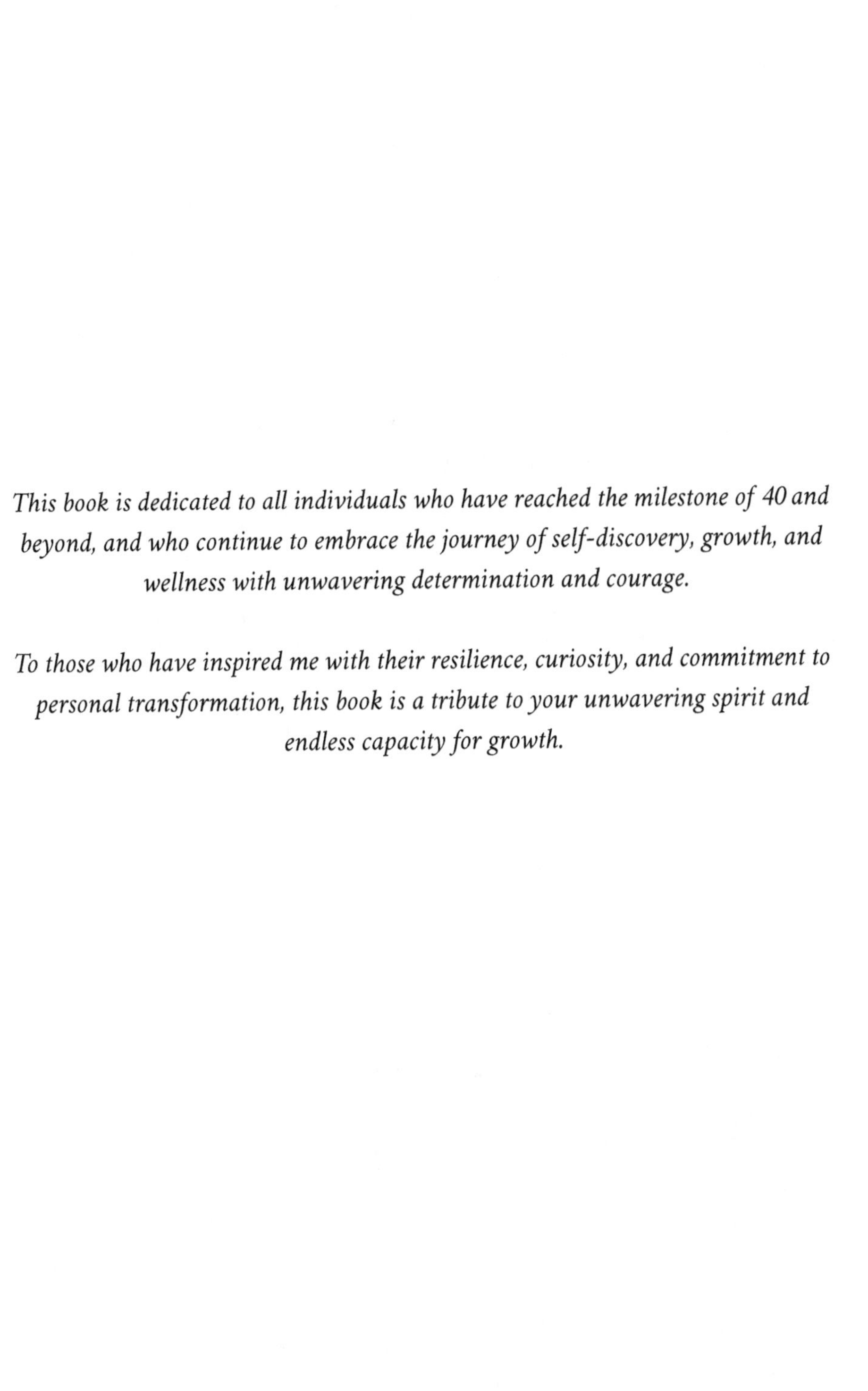

This book is dedicated to all individuals who have reached the milestone of 40 and beyond, and who continue to embrace the journey of self-discovery, growth, and wellness with unwavering determination and courage.

To those who have inspired me with their resilience, curiosity, and commitment to personal transformation, this book is a tribute to your unwavering spirit and endless capacity for growth.

Age is not a barrier to wellness; it is an opportunity to redefined it

— Celia C. Hisey

Contents

Preface

As we age, our body undergoes significant changes, and maintaining optimal health becomes increasingly crucial. In recent years, intermittent fasting has gained immense popularity as a lifestyle approach that can offer remarkable health benefits. "Wellness Beyond 40" is a comprehensive guide designed for individuals navigating the vibrant years beyond 40. This book provides a structured 21-day plan tailored specifically for men and women to embrace intermittent fasting as a tool for achieving sustainable wellness.

The book draws upon the latest scientific research and practical insights to equip you with the knowledge and support needed to thrive on your wellness journey. The 21-day plan outlined in the book is meticulously crafted with actionable strategies to seamlessly incorporate fasting into your daily routine to help you achieve your health goals.

The book explores the fundamentals of intermittent fasting, including understanding the various fasting protocols, debunking common myths, navigating potential challenges, and optimizing your results. Each chapter is designed to empower you with the knowledge and support needed to embrace intermittent fasting as a lifestyle approach for achieving optimal health.

In addition to the 21-day plan, the book provides a comprehensive overview of the science behind intermittent fasting. You will learn about the physiological and metabolic changes that occur during fasting and how they can benefit your health. The book also offers guidance on how to create a personalized fasting plan that fits your unique needs and lifestyle.

Ultimately, this book is a testament to the transformative power of self-care and the boundless potential that lies within each of us to reclaim our health and vitality. By embarking on this transformative journey, you can unlock the full potential of your body and mind. Thank you for choosing "Wellness Beyond 40" as your guide to better health.

1

Chapter 1

Understanding Intermittent Fasting (IF)

1.1 What is Intermittent Fasting?

Intermittent fasting, which can also be termed as IF, exploits the capacity of the body to access a fasting state, and uses metabolic flexibility in directing the body to use stored energy. In fasting procedures, the human insulin levels fall down stimulating the body to go from glucose metabolism to fat-burning. This metabolic change is expected to lead to weight loss and other health advantages.

Other than benefits related to weight loss, intermittent fasting has been linked to other benefits such as improved insulin sensitivity and lowered inflammation levels and increased brain function. Some studies indicate a potential health benefit to the heart, because blood pressure and cholesterol levels are reduced.

It is worth mentioning that intermittent fasting is not for all people, and subjective reactions appear. The aging process may be determined by the age; health conditions; lifestyle, and other factors should be taken into account as well. Also, balanced and healthy diets during ingestion windows must be practiced in order to ensure good overall health.

One is always advised to seek advice from a health practitioner before stepping into the fasting journey, and especially for those individuals who are dealing with underlying health issues. The solution, in essence, is to find an effective and customized solution that fits health goals and lifestyle properly for midlife adults (men and women above the age of 40).

1.2 Denying the Myths of Fasting

When discussing the problems of intermittent fasting for men and women over 40 years old, it is necessary to address numerous fallacies and several myths that abound concerning this lifestyle that needs to be clarified. This is why it allows us to convey the accurate data and improve awareness of the pros and cons of practicing IF. The approach has gained much popularity in recent trends but there are doubts that still remain unanswered pertaining to whether it is applied on the adult aged population. It is, therefore, necessary to de-stigmatize these baseless beliefs and help clear any ambiguity that may still prevail. Now, let us take a short overview of the myths of intermittent fasting.

1. Myth: "Intermittent Fasting Decreases the Metabolic Rate of Older Individuals"

Intermittent fasting can improve metabolism by improving the body's utilization of stored energy. Research suggests that it does not result in a major decrease in metabolic rate.

2. Myth: "Seniors Experience Nutrient Deficiencies When Fasting Intermittent Fasting"

This is not true because, when done properly, IF can give important nutrients at designated meal hours. Consuming a meal that is balanced in nutrients is crucial for meeting one's nutritional needs.

3. Myth: "Aging Populations Will Encounter Heightened Malnutrition and Irritability"

Intermittent fasting is typically linked to reduced appetite over a longer period. By getting into a fasting habit gradually, any early pain may be lessened.

4. Myth: "Older Adults Should Not Be Allowed to Fast Due to Medication Interactions"

To explain, fasting may be properly integrated into a pharmacological routine if the right medical care is offered. Consulting with healthcare providers is important for personalized care.

5. Myth: "As You Age, You Can't Lose Weight with Intermittent Fasting"

Research shows that IF, which increases fat loss while keeping lean muscle mass, can aid persons over 40 in controlling their weight.

6. Myth: "Fasting Isn't Good for Bone Health in Older Adults"

To be clear, regular movement and ingesting appropriate calcium at mealtimes can improve bone health. Fasting does not generally have a bad effect on bone health.

7. Myth: "Older Women Cannot Fast Due to Hormonal Changes"

To be clear, women normally go through menopause with differences in their hormones. One result of intermittent fasting that might be useful at this time of life is better insulin sensitivity.

8. Myth: "Elderly People Who Fast Experience Severe Muscle Loss"

When paired with physical exercise and a proper protein diet, intermittent fasting can help elderly people keep their muscle mass.

9. Myth: "Seniors Need to Eat Often to Maintain Energy Levels"

To be clear, IF may promote metabolic flexibility, which could help the body use stored fat and glucose more effectively for energy and lead to longer bursts of energy.

10. Myth: "Fasting is Problematic for Midlife Adults Suffering from Chronic Health Issues"

With the appropriate medical advice from proper medical experts, intermittent fasting can work with many health conditions. It could even provide advantages with conditions such as type 2 diabetes and cardiovascular health control.

11. Myth: "It is best that the midlife adults take small meals all through the day as a way to having an optimum health condition"

Substantiating the daily regime of small meals and addressing the idea of some selected period interval, one can say that a well-arranged and quality feeding during specific windows may be enough for sustaining health and nutrition.

12. Myth: "Fastening has a negative impact on cognitive functioning in aged individuals"

Other research indicates that intermittent fasting may improve brain function, increasing neural plasticity and lowering the possibility of age-related neurodegenerative disease.

13. Myth: "Regardless of Men and Women, Intermittent Fasting Produces a Similar Effect Above the Age of 40"

There could be hormone-based gender-specific differences that affect responses to intermittent fasting. Fine-tuning fasting methods to accommodate such disparities can, in turn, maximize results not only for women but also for men above 40.

These myths and clarifications help to create a clearer picture of intermittent fasting, as the nuanced understanding of this approach for older persons is implemented on these grounds.

1.3 Benefits of Intermittent Fasting for Women Over 40

1. Balance of Hormones: Irregular eating might uphold hormonal equilibrium, particularly for midlife women, which are women above age 40, managing conditions like Polycystic Ovary Syndrome (PCOS). It can assist with controlling insulin levels and further develop awareness, decidedly working on hormonal well-being.

2. Weight Management: Fasting can help people lose weight by cutting calories. Women, even above the age of 40, may also gain a healthier body composition by burning more fat during fasting while maintaining lean muscle mass.

3. Improved Insulin Sensitivity: Irregular fasting further develops insulin awareness, significant for midlife women in keeping ordinary glucose levels. People who are at risk for or already have type 2 diabetes may benefit most from this.

4. Clarity of Thought: Women's mental clarity and brain function may benefit from fasting. The brain prefers to use the ketone bodies produced during fasting as a source of energy.

5.Heart Health: Intermittent fasting has shown guarantee in working on cardiovascular well-being for midlife women by bringing down risk factors, for example, cholesterol levels, circulatory strain, and irritation.

6. Diminished Chance of Breast Cancer: By altering hormone levels and insulin sensitivity, intermittent fasting may reduce the risk of breast cancer, according to some studies.

7. Anti-Aging and Cellular Repair: Autophagy is encouraged and cellular repair mechanisms are sparked by fasting, possibly slowing down aging and reducing cellular oxidative stress.

8. Further developed Temperament and Mental Well-being: A few women report better joy and mental prosperity during irregular fasting, which could be connected to the constructive outcomes of synapses and hormonal control.

9. Life span Benefits: By promoting cellular health, reducing inflammation, and supporting general well-being, intermittent fasting has been linked to potential longevity benefits. This can be especially crucial for women as they age.

10. Bone Health: intermittent fasting, when matched with a supplement rich eating regimen, can add to bone well-being by expanding calcium admission and mineralization, significant for midlife women's bone thickness, particularly post-menopause.

11. Diminished Inflammation: Fasting might assist with bringing down irritation in the body, a variable connected to various constant illnesses. Women may benefit from this because chronic inflammation is linked to arthritis and autoimmune diseases.

12. Enhanced Fat Absorption: IF urges the body to use fat for energy, helping women in fat digestion and potentially supporting weight reduction endeavors proficiently.

13. Healthier Skin: By reducing oxidative stress and inflammation, fasting may help maintain healthy skin. A few women report changes in skin and diminished indications of maturing with sporadic fasting.

14. Better Quality Sleep: Laying out a normal eating window through IF could emphatically influence circadian rhythms, conceivably prompting better rest quality for midlife women.

15. Adjusted Glucose Levels: Intermittent fasting can assist with balancing

out glucose levels in midlife women, bringing down the opportunity of insulin obstruction and type 2 diabetes.

16. Autophagy Enhanced: During fasting, the cellular process of autophagy, which removes damaged cells, is encouraged, possibly assisting women in the prevention of age-related diseases.

17. Boosts Healthful Reproduction: By promoting hormone balance, intermittent fasting may help women with fertility issues or irregular menstrual cycles improve their reproductive health.

18. Enhanced Energy Levels: A few women report higher energy levels during fasting times, which could be connected to better mitochondrial capability and energy utilization.

It's important to remember that different people react differently to intermittent fasting, so it's a good idea to talk to a doctor, especially if you're a woman who has specific health problems or conditions.

1.4 Benefits of Intermittent Fasting for Men Over 40

1. Weight Loss and Fat Reduction: By causing a calorie shortage during fasting windows, IF helps people lose weight by lowering body fat while keeping lean muscle mass.

2. Muscle Preservation and Growth: When paired with resistance training, fasting help muscles stay healthy and grow by increasing the production of human growth hormone and creating an environment that is good for building muscle.

3. Better Insulin Sensitivity: By making the body better at responding to glucose, intermittent fasting raises insulin sensitivity and lowers the risk of insulin resistance and type 2 diabetes.

4. Better cardiovascular health: Fasting may be good for your heart by dropping your blood pressure, cholesterol, and inflammation, which can help lower your risk of getting heart disease.

5. Cognitive Function and Mental Clarity: Intermittent fasting may improve cognitive function and mental clarity, possibly improving attention, concentration, and general brain health.

6. Hormonal Optimization: IF causes hormonal changes, including higher production of norepinephrine and human growth hormone, boosting fat metabolism and muscle retention.

7. Cellular Repair and Longevity: IF triggers cellular repair mechanisms, possibly increasing lifespan by lowering oxidative stress and supporting overall cellular health even in men above 40.

8. Reduced Inflammation: Intermittent fasting has anti-inflammatory benefits, which can help alleviate chronic inflammation linked to different illnesses and conditions common in midlife men.

9. Improved Metabolic Health: IF positively impacts metabolic markers, such as lowering triglycerides and improving lipid profiles, adding to better general metabolic health.

10. Simplicity and Convenience: Intermittent fasting is simple to adopt, offering a handy and manageable approach to health and wellness for men with busy lives.

11. Higher Levels of Testosterone: An important and growth-promoting hormone for midlife men's reproductive and general health, testosterone levels may be positively impacted by intermittent fasting.

12. Enhanced Energy Efficiency: Fasting improves energy usage and may

lessen symptoms of exhaustion by encouraging the body to consume fat that has been stored as fuel.

13. Helps Maintain Prostate Health: According to certain research, men who fast on and off may be less likely to experience problems connected to their prostates.

14. Increased Sports Efficiency: By maximizing nutrition timing and increasing metabolic flexibility, intermittent fasting in conjunction with deliberate meal planning has the potential to improve athletic performance.

15. Higher Quality Sleep: Men may have better quality sleep if they can optimize their circadian rhythms by sometimes fasting and establishing regular eating periods.

16. Decreased Type 2 Diabetes Risk: By promoting healthy blood sugar levels and increasing insulin sensitivity, intermittent fasting can reduce the incidence of type 2 diabetes.

17. Increased Immune Response: Fasting may promote autophagy, which is the elimination of damaged cells from the body, strengthening the immune system and maybe lowering the risk of disease.

18. Increase in Joint Health: Intermittent fasting improves joint health; this is because it lowers inflammation and improves overall metabolic health.

19. Good Effect on Emotion: Fasting intermittently can improve mental health and happiness by encouraging self-control and awareness when eating.

20. Suggested Long-Term Health Behaviors: Men's long-term health and well-being are enhanced by intermittent fasting, which promotes the formation of enduring and healthful eating habits.

These advantages offer a thorough grasp of the ways that intermittent fasting might improve several facets of midlife men's health. As with any lifestyle modification, it's crucial to approach intermittent fasting with awareness for specific medical concerns and, if necessary, seek medical counsel.

1.5 Who Should Not Fast?

Some people should approach intermittent fasting cautiously or not at all, as it may not be suited for them. Before commencing intermittent fasting, persons who come into the following categories should talk with a healthcare provider:

1. People Who Have Eating Disorders: Periodic fasting has the potential to create or aggravate eating disorders like bulimia or anorexia. Restrictive eating habits should be avoided by persons who have a history of these disorders.

2. Women Who Are Pregnant or Nursing: Consistent dietary intake is required for the development of the fetus and baby in pregnant and nursing moms. It's probable that intermittent fasting won't offer adequate nourishment throughout important growth periods.

3. People with a Medical Background or Present Illnesses: Particular dietary choices may be important for particular medical problems, such as diabetes, metabolic disorders, or cardiovascular diseases. Seeking assistance from a medical specialist is crucial to assure safety.

4. People Who Worry About Being Underweight or Low Body Weight: Unintentional weight loss could arise from intermittent fasting. People who are already underweight or who struggle with their weight should avoid from acts that can damage their health even more.

5. Youngsters and Teenagers: A continuous supply of nutrients is required for the growth and development of young individuals. Fasting intermittently

might not offer adequate nourishment throughout important developmental phases.

6. People with a Past Hypoglycemia: Low blood sugar levels brought on by intermittent fasting may make hypoglycemia symptoms worse. People who have suffered hypoglycemia in the past ought to consult with a medical specialist before starting intermittent fasting.

7. Persons Suffering from Prolonged Stress or Cortisol Imbalance: The stress hormone cortisol may rise during intermittent fasting. People who now have cortisol imbalances or chronic stress should take care not to place themselves in more stress situations.

8. Medication Users: For best absorption and efficacy, some medications may need to be taken on a regular basis when eating. It is advisable to change fasting regimens under a doctor's supervision when taking drugs.

9. People with a Past History of Digestive Problems: For patients who suffer from gastrointestinal issues such acid reflux, Irritable Bowel Syndrome (IBS), or inflammatory bowel infections, intermittent fasting may make their symptoms worse.

10. Individuals with Compromised Immune System: People with compromised immune systems might not benefit from the immune system modifications brought on by fasting. This covers persons who have recently had surgery or autoimmune illnesses.

11. Seniors with Frailty Concerns: Seniors experiencing frailty or those at risk of malnutrition may struggle to achieve their nutritional demands during intermittent fasting, thereby jeopardizing their health.

12. People with a History of Migraines: Intermittent fasting may provoke migraines or aggravate existing disorders in certain individuals. Those prone

to migraines should be cautious and watch their responses.

13. Individuals with Sleep Disorders: Irregular eating patterns linked with intermittent fasting may affect sleep-wake cycles. People with sleep problems or those prone to sleep disruptions should evaluate the possible influence on their sleep quality.

14. Those having a History of Gallbladder Issues: Intermittent fasting can lead to alterations in bile production and flow, possibly influencing those with a history of gallbladder disorders. Consultation with a healthcare expert is advisable.

15. People Engaging in Intense Physical Training or Athletes in Competitive Seasons: Intermittent fasting may impact performance in severe physical activity. Athletes in competitive seasons or persons involved in high-intensity training should carefully assess the possible influence on their energy levels and recuperation.

Individuals falling within these categories should contact with a healthcare practitioner before going on intermittent fasting. Personalized counsel ensures that any dietary adjustments fit with individual health needs and goals.

It's vital to talk with a healthcare physician before commencing any fasting program, particularly for people who come into these categories. Individualized instruction assures that intermittent fasting is in accordance with specific health requirements and aspirations.

2

Chapter 2

Getting Started

2.1 Types of Intermittent Fasting

These represent a diverse range of intermittent fasting approaches, offering flexibility for individuals to choose based on their preferences and health goals.

2.1.1 16/8 Method (Time-Restricted Eating)

This is also known as Time-Restricted Eating, entails devoting specific times throughout the day to eating and fasting. This is the standard technique:

1. Select Your Eating Window: Settle on a 8-hour timeframe during the day to eat the entirety of your caloric admission. Meal times are typically from 1:00 p.m. to 9:30 p.m. or from 12:00 p.m. to 8:00 p.m.

2. Identify Your Fasting Period: Avoid eating for the next sixteen hours. For some individuals, this period is more straightforward to endure since it incorporates rest.

3. Stay hydrated: During the fasting time frame, remain hydrated and control your craving by drinking water, home-made teas, or dark espresso.

4. Begin Gradually: If you have never intermittently fasted before, you might want to gradually extend your fasting period. At the point when you get to the 16-hour fasting window, begin with a 12-hour fast and progressively broaden it.

5. Select Supplement Thick Foods: To ensure you meet your dietary prerequisites, focus on eating adjusted, supplement thick foods during your eating window.

6. Take Care of Your Body: Pay attention to your body's signals of hunger and fullness. It's important to eat enough during the eating window to meet your energy needs.

7. Keep your word: To assist your body with becoming used to the propensity, try to keep a reliable eating and fasting plan.

8. Incorporate into a healthy way of life: The best outcomes from intermittent fasting come from a fair, empowering way of life that incorporates ordinary activity and a balanced eating routine.

9. Consider exercising during the fasting window: Certain individuals decide to plan their activities during their fasting period to exploit potential benefits like expanded fat consuming.

10. Keep an eye on your health: Focus on how the 16/8 strategy influences your body. If you have any concerns or negative effects, talk to a doctor.

Realize that different people may respond to intermittent fasting differently. However it probably won't be the most ideal choice for everybody, the 16/8 Method is a popular and versatile strategy. Prior to beginning any sort of fasting routine, you genuinely should talk with a medical services proficient in the event that you have any previous medical issue.

2.1.2 5:2 Diet (Modified Fasting)

The second type of fasting is 5:2 Diet – Modified Fasting, which is an intermittent fasting practice that involves a dietary pattern where alternate days are days of normal eating and days of significant calorie restriction.

1. Choose Fasting Days: Choose two days from the entire week and do not let them be consecutive to make the fasting days. These are days of great abstinence from calorie consumption.

2. On all other five days of the week, just eat a normal balanced diet but with moderate calorie restrictions.

3. During fasting, do not exceed 500-600 calories per each day. This maly be done by having smaller meals enriched with nutrients.

4. Spread Caloric Intake: Share out the rationed calorie consumption over the fasting day, between small meals. This assists in suppressing the urge to eat throughout the day.

5. Here, select food that has the crucial nutrients but few calories. Choose lean proteins, vegetables, and healthy fats-based foods.

6. Stay Hydrated: On fast days, make sure you drink plenty of water, herbal teas or any other non-caloric beverages to help in hydration and to assist in managing hunger.

7. Select fasting days that will match your work/lifestyle. Weekdays also find preference among some people while weekends stand out for others.

8. Monitor Physical Activity: It would be worth your while to modify your workout schedule as appropriate fasting days on the basis of your levels of energy. In low-calorie days, light or moderate activities are more likely to be appropriate.

9. Be Consistent: For the sake of assimilation, try to obey uniformity for your fasting and non-fasting days.

If you are too exhausted or sick, you need to reconsider the way of doing this or see a doctor.

2.1.3 Alternate-Day Fasting

Alternate-Day Fasting is a type of intermittent fasting in which days of typical eating are alternated with days of severe calorie restriction or full fasting. Here is an identified clarification of how Alternate-Day Fasting is typically done:

1. Select the days you need to fast: Choose which days you want to fast. You might choose to fast, for example, when at regular intervals or on specific working days.

2. Define the Fasting Schedule: Lay out the number of calories that should be tried on fasting days. While certain structures call for complete fasting, others might allow a limited calorie consumption (like 500-600 calories).

3. Eat Ordinarily on Non-Fasting Days: On non-fasting days, consume a typical, well-balanced diet without strict calorie restrictions. Ensure you are getting the sustenance you expect nowadays.

4. Spread Caloric Admission on Fasting Days: To assist with controlling craving, spread out the calories you consume on fasting days into short, supplement thick dinners over the course of the day.

5.   Remain Hydrated: On fasting days, stay hydrated and assist with controlling your craving by drinking lots of water, home-made teas, or other non-caloric fluids.

6. Adjust Exercise Schedule: Consider altering your workout schedule in response to your energy levels. On days when you are fasting, hcaptivating in light or moderate activity could be better.

7. Maintain a close eye on your mental and physical health: See how your body responds to fasting on rotating days. In the event that you experience the ill effects of serious weariness, dizziness, or opposite aftereffects, re-examine the technique or talk with a health professional.j.

8. Be Consistent: Keep the fasting and non-fasting plan predictable so your body can become accustomed to the new propensity.

9. Select a Methodology that Fits You: There are a few ways to deal with substitute day fasting; pick the one that best accommodates your preferences and lifestyle. Some people can choose to eat fewer calories than others on days when they fast.

10. Think about the sustainability over the long term: Decide if Alternate-8Day Fasting is a long haul, manageable technique for you. Any eating routine arrangement that is effective should be economical.

It's memorable that not every person is ideal for substitute day fasting. Prior to starting any fasting program, anybody with previous well-being illnesses or concerns ought to talk with a medical services supplier. Fulfilling wholesome needs likewise requires focusing on supplement thick dinners on both fasting and non-fasting days.

2.1.4 Eat-Stop-Eat

A few of 24-hour diets every week are crucial for the Eat-Stop-Eat intermittent fasting technique. This is an identified clarification of how Eat-Stop-Eat is typically done:

1. Select Fasting Period: Choose which days of the week you will fast, if any. You may, for instance, opt to fast from supper one day until dinner the following.

2. Begin and End the Fast: On the specified day, begin the fast after supper and end it simultaneously the following day. Consequently, a complete 24-hour fast is observed.

3. Remain Hydrated: All during the fasting stage, maintain hydrated and regulate your appetite by drinking plenty of water, home-made teas, or other non-caloric fluids.

4. Continue Customary Eating: Return to your usual eating regimen when the fasting time is ended. There are no special food needs during non-fasting times.

5. Select the Fitting Time: Select fasting days as per your daily practice and lifestyle. For improved adherence, several individuals find it easy to start the fast after dinner.

6. Watch out for your bodily and psychological wellness: Notice your body's response to the Eat-Stop-Eat convention. In the event that you suffer the bad consequences of outrageous fatigue, dazedness, or some other undesirable incidental effects, mull over the system or see a professional.

7. Adjust Exercise Schedule: Consider adjusting your exercise schedule for agreement with your energy levels when fasting. Taking part in mild or

direct activities might be preferable.

8. Steady Adaptation: On the off chance that you've never abstained, think starting with a solitary 24-hour fast every week and progressing progressively up to two times per week as your body transforms.

9. The key is consistency: Keep to your fasting schedule dependably so your body may develop accustomed to it.

10. Pay attention to Your Body: Know about your body's indicators of craving and fullness. To meet your dietary demands, it's crucial that you consume enough during non-fasting periods.

2.1.5 Warrior Diet

The Warrior Diet is a intermittent fasting approach that involves eating humble parts of new leafy foods during the day and requiring one significant dinner around evening time inside a 4-hour eating window. Here is a bit-by-bit guidance on how the Warrior Diet regimen is ordinarily done:

1. Daytime Undereating: During the daytime, center around ingesting little portions of fresh foods grown from the ground. These foods are much of the time low in calories yet high in supplements.

2. Stay Hydrated: Hydrate, natural teas, or other non-caloric fluids over the course of the day to keep hydrated and assist with controlling appetite.

3. Get ready for the dinner party: As the day proceeds, expect your significant dinner at night. This will be the ideal opportunity for your bigger, more significant banquet.

4. 4-Hour Eating Window: During a 4-hour eating window at night, partake

in your primary dinner. This lunch can incorporate a scope of dinners, including proteins, solid fats, and carbs.

5. Concentrate on foods high in nutrients: To ensure that you meet your daily nutritional requirements for the evening meal, choose meals that are high in nutrients. Incorporate an assortment of food classifications for a decent dinner.

6. Eat an Assortment of meals: Utilize the night blowout to eat different dinners that you could have been longing for during the day. The dish might taste better as a result of this.

7. Pay attention to Your Body: Focus on your body's appetite and fullness signs. It's pivotal to eat enough at the night banquet to suit your wholesome desires.

8. Change Your Way of Life: Adjust the Warrior Diet to your way of life and tastes. You might pick specific days for this eating design or apply it constantly over time.

9. Consistency is Key: Keep up with consistency with the Warrior Diet regimen to assist your body with acclimating to the program.

10. Monitor Physical and Mental Well-Being: Focus on how your body answers the Warrior Diet. In the event that you experience any unsafe impacts, rethink the technique or talk with a health professionalr.

2.1.6 One Meal a Day (OMAD)

The One Meal a Day (OMAD) approach is a type of intermittent fasting wherein individuals eat all of their day-to-day caloric admission at one dinner, once in a while inside a one-hour time span. Here is a full aide on the typical advances engaged with performing OMAD:

1. Select Your Supper time Window: Settle on a specific window of time for your one dinner consistently. A one-hour eating window or a four-hour supper window are normal substitutions.

2. Evaluate the Fasting Period: The remainder of the day is viewed as the Fasting Period. Ordinarily, this is a 23-hour time, including rest, for fasting.

3. Remain Hydrated: All through the fasting stage, remain hydrated and control your craving by taking lots of water, home-made teas, or other non-caloric beverages.

4. Begin Little and Gradual: In the event that you are new to IF or OMAD, consider expanding your eating window from the start and gradually bringing it down as your body changes.

5. Arrange a Meal High in Nutrients: Ensure your food is adjusted and high in nutrients since you are eating every one of the calories you want for the day without a moment's delay. Integrate a scope of nutrition types, including carbs, great fats, and proteins.

6. Incorporate an Assortment of Meals: Make the most of the opportunity to eat a scope of dinners that meet your dietary necessities.

7. Focus on Your Body: During your dinner, focus on your body's indications of craving and totality. Eating sufficient food to meet your everyday well-being needs is significant.

8. Conform to Your Lifestyle: Alter OMAD to fit with your timetable and lifestyle. You might design your everyday dinner at a particular time or change it in light of how occupied you are that day.

9. Watch out for Your Physical and Mental Health: See how your body answers OMAD. On the off chance that you experience any bad secondary

effects, reconsider the seeking help from an expert.

10. Consistency is Key: Keep doing OMAD consistently with the goal that your body can become used to the timetable.

2.1.7 The 12-Hour Fast

A simple way to deal with intermittent fasting is the 12-Hour Fast, which involves fasting for 12 hours and eating inside that equivalent window of time. This is a regular bit-by-bit plan for completing the 12-hour fast:

1. Select Your Fasting Window: We should envision you wish to fast for 12 hours. You might choose to fast, for example, from 7:00 PM to 7:00 AM or some other 12-hour window that works with your everyday routine.

2. Begin with an Early supper: Have an early dinner to begin your fasting window. This gives a more drawn out time of fasting past to the following day's meal.

3. Remain Hydrated: During the fasting time frame, stay hydrated and limit your yearning by drinking water, natural teas, or other non-caloric refreshments.

4. Continuous Adaptation: In the event that you're not knowledgeable about IF, you should begin with a lower window of time (say, 10 hours) and move gradually as long as 12 hours as your body becomes adjusted to it.

5. Pick Food varieties High in Supplements: Make an endeavor to have adjusted, supplement thick dinners during the ideal opportunity for eating. A variety of wholesome classes, including proteins, starches, and sound fats, ought to be provided.

6. Incorporate Breakfast: In the event that you would like to break your fast

with a nutritious meal, make arrangements to do as such. Your digestion might get a lift from this for the afternoon.

7. Reliable Timing: Make an endeavor to keep your everyday eating and fasting windows at similar timings. This can help in your body's adaption to the plan.

8. Track Physical and Mental Welfare: Notice your body's response to the 12-Hour fast. Assuming you experience any awful effects, re-examine the technique or look for professional guidance.

9. Adjust to Your Lifestyle: Adjust the 12-Hour Fast to accommodate your preferences and lifestyle. A movable technique functions admirably with a scope of schedules.

10. Steady Changes: Give your body time to adjust to the time of fasting. Focus on your body's signs of appetite and completion, and adjust as the need should arise.

2.1.8 Crescendo Fasting

An intermittent fasting technique called Crescendo Fasting involves inconsistent fasting on non-back to back days. This is an ordinary bit-by-bit guideline for finishing Crescendo Fasting:

1. Select Fasting Days: Lay out a fast for a few non-sequential days every week. You might decide to fast, for example, on Mondays, Wednesdays, and Fridays.

2. Decide Fasting Duration: Lay out how long each fasting day will be. While there are numerous varieties, a common technique is to fast for around 12 to 16 hours.

3. Progressive Onset: On the off chance that you're curious about intermittent fasting, ponder lessening the length of the fast from the beginning and afterward logically broadening it as your body changes. For example, start with a 12-hour fast and move gradually up to a 16-hour fast.

4. Remain Hydrated: All through the fasting period, stay hydrated and control your craving by drinking water, natural teas, or other non-caloric fluids.

5. Alter exercise Schedule: On days when you are fasting, consider changing your exercise plan for agreement with how fiery you are. Taking part in light or direct activities can be better.

6. Select Food sources High in Supplements: When you fast, focus on eating foods that are high in supplements. A scope of dietary classes, including proteins, carbs, and sound fats, ought to be incorporated.

7. Non-Fasting Days: Eat a normal, even eating regimen without thorough calorie constraints on non-fasting days. Ensure you are getting the sustenance you expect.

8. Pay attention to Your Body: Focus on the signs that your body sends whether it is ravenous or full. To accomplish your healthful requests, you must consume enough during non-fasting periods.

9. Solidness is Key: Stick to the Crescendo Fasting plan reliably with the goal that your body can become accustomed to the new example.

10. Watch out for Your Physical and Mental Health: See how your body responds to Crescendo Fasting. Assuming you experience any adverse consequences, rethink the procedure or seek help from and expert.

2.1.9 Spontaneous Meal Skipping

A flexible method of intermittent fasting called "Spontaneous Meal Skipping" enables participants to skip meals whenever it's convenient for them, taking into account their daily schedules and degree of hunger. This is a how-to guide for executing spontaneous meal skipping:

1. Pay Attention to Your Body: Observe the signals your body sends whether it is hungry or full. Try missing a certain supper if you're not feeling particularly hungry at that time.

2. No Tight Timetable: Unlike other forms of intermittent fasting, there is no set schedule for spontaneous meal skipping. It is determined by your daily mood.

3. Remain Hydrated: When skipping meals, stay hydrated by consuming water, herbal teas, or other non-caloric beverages.

4. Eat When Hungry: Consume a nutritious meal as soon as you feel hungry. The kinds of meals you can consume are unlimited.

5. Gradual Adaptation: If you're not used to skipping meals on the spur of the moment, begin slowly. Before introducing it more often, skip a meal now and again to observe how your body responds.

6. Select Meals You Can Skip: It's simple for some people to skip meals, such as lunch or breakfast. Select a lunchtime that corresponds with your typical eating pattern.

7. Adjust to Lifestyle: Modify your way of life to accommodate spontaneous meal skipping. It's an adaptable approach that can be tailored to suit various schedules and preferences.

8. Track Physical and Mental Welfare: Observe your body's reaction to unplanned meal skipping. If you encounter any negative consequences, re-evaluate the procedure or see a health professional.

9. No Caloric limit: Spontaneous meal skipping has no severe calorie restriction. Eating when hungry and skipping meals when not is the main focus.

10. Consistency is Key: Although there isn't a rigid timetable, your body will adjust to this adaptable strategy if you maintain some regularity when skipping meals on the spur of the moment.

2.1.10 Extended Fasting (24 Hours or More)

A high level sort of intermittent fasting is classified "Extended Fasting," which includes fasting for 24 hours or longer at a time. This is a guide making sense of the standard system for Extended Fasting:

1. Select Fasting Duration: Pick how long you need to keep your drawn out fast going. Choices like 24, 36, 48, or even 72 hours are oftentimes picked. Stretched out diets should be painstakingly arranged and noticed.

2. Steady Adaptation: In the event that you're curious about drawn out fasting, contemplate extending it gradually from the beginning and perceiving how your body changes. This empowers you to understand the responses of your body.

3. Remain Hydrated: To remain hydrated during the fast, take lots of water. To assist with hydration, you can likewise drink natural tea.

4. Keep away from Caloric Intake: During the fasting stage, abstain from taking any calories. A significant diminishing in calorie utilization is important for delayed fasting.

5. Monitor Energy Levels: All through the fast, watch out for your overall prosperity and level of energy. Long-term fasting might affect energy levels and cause mental lucidity in specific people.

7. Breaking the Fast: Arrange your fast breaking system. For your most memorable dinner, decide for supplement thick meals; begin with a more modest piece and move gradually up to a standard dinner size.

8. Select a Safe Environment: Ensure you are in a safe setting while noticing a drawn out fast, especially in the event that you are approaching your customary business. At the point when your body advises you to unwind, do as such.

9. Talk with a Professional: Prior to attempting extended fasting, particularly for periods longer than 24 hours, it is suggested that you talk with a medical care expert on the off chance that you have any previous health issues.

10. Introduce food sources step-by-step following a delayed fast. To forestall straining your stomach related framework, begin with low-volume, promptly processed foods.

2.1.11 Spontaneous Eating Windows

With the Spontaneous Eating Windows method of intermittent fasting, people select various meal windows on different days according to their schedules or personal preferences. Here's a guide explaining the standard procedure for Spontaneous Eating Windows:

1. Pay Attention to Your Body: Pay attention to how hungry and how energetic your body is feeling. When it fits with your daily schedule or when you are naturally hungry, pick a time to eat.

2. No Fixed Schedule: Spontaneous Eating Windows provide for flexibility,

in contrast to scheduled intermittent fasting approaches. The beginning and ending times of your dining window are not set.

3. Remain Hydrated: To stay hydrated, sip on water, herbal teas, or other non-caloric drinks when you're not eating.

4. Adjust to Daily Schedule: Select meal times that coincide with your everyday activity. For instance, your window for eating may be later in the day if you're more busy in the evening.

5. Include Foods High in Nutrients: When you do eat, make sure your meals are balanced and high in nutrients. A range of dietary categories, including proteins, carbs, and healthy fats, should be included.

6. Adjust Based on Lifestyle: Modify your eating schedule in accordance with your way of living. You may find that a shorter eating window works better on certain days and that a longer window works better on others.

7. No Limit on Calories: When using Spontaneous Eating Windows, there is no rigorous calorie control. Eating at the moment of hunger and timing meals according to your body's natural rhythm are the main points of attention.

8. Keep an Eye on Your Physical and Mental Health: Observe how your body reacts to unplanned Meals. If you encounter any negative consequences, think about changing the strategy or seeking advice from a medical expert.

9. Choose Foods Mindfully: Throughout your eating windows, choose your foods carefully. If you want to be sure you are getting enough nutrients, choose whole, unprocessed meals.

10. Consistency in Flexibility: Although you can choose your eating windows freely, your body will adjust to this impromptu method if you keep some

consistency in your overall time.

2.1.12 The 14/10 Method

An unassuming kind of intermittent fasting, the 14/10 method (at times called the 14-hour fast) substitutes a 10-hour eating window with a 14-hour fasting window.

1. Make Your Fasting and Eating Windows: Settle on a 14-hour fasting window and a 10-hour eating window. Fasting from 7:00 PM to 9:00 AM the following day is a well known decision.

2. Progressive Adaptation: In the event that you're curious about intermittent fasting, consider decreasing the span of your fasting window from the outset and afterward continuously protracting it. For example, when your body changes, you might start with a 12-hour fast and move gradually up to a 14-hour one.

3. Remain Hydrated: During the fasting stage, stay hydrated and control your craving by drinking water, natural teas, or other non-caloric fluids.

4. Fit in with Your Schedule: Select a fasting window that fits with your normal daily practice. While certain people decide to start their fast in the first part of the day, others observe that beginning at night is more functional.

5. Reliable Timing: Try to keep your everyday eating and fasting windows at similar times. This can support your body's transformation to the timetable.

6. Select Food sources High in Supplements: Try to consume adjusted, supplement thick food over the course of the ideal opportunity for eating. A scope of dietary classes, including proteins, carbs, and solid fats, ought to be incorporated.

7. Incorporate Breakfast: In the event that you love breakfast, ensure this dinner is remembered for your eating window.

8. Track Physical and Mental Welfare: Notice your body's response to the 14/10 strategy. In the event that you experience any unfortunate results, consider changing the technique or looking for advice from an health professional.

9. Slow Adjustments: Give your body time to become used to the fasting period. Focus on your body's signs of yearning and fullness, and adjust as needs be.

10. Consistency is Key: Follow the 14/10 Strategy reliably with the goal that your body can become used to the timetable.

2.1.13 Fasting Mimicking Diet (FMD)

A sort of dietary mediation called the Fasting Mimicking Diet (FMD) plans to duplicate the advantages of fasting while offering some food. Typically, a pattern of supplement thick, low-calorie meal is involved. This is the way to direct your Fasting Mimicking Diet:

1. Select Fasting Period: Decide how long your FMD cycle will endure. A 5-day cycle is a run of the mill technique, but there are more choices. The FMD is much of the time controlled consistently, maybe one time each month or like clockwork.

2. Talk with a Professional: Ensure the FMD is in accordance with your well-being targets by talking with an enlisted dietitian or medical care proficient prior to starting, particularly to follow it for quite a while.

3. Calorie Restriction: Keep your day-to-day calorie consumption during the fasting imitating days inside a specific reach, frequently somewhere in

the range of 40 and 60 percent of your expectation. This calorie limitation is one of the FMD's fundamental elements.

4. High-Supplement Meals: Ensure your meal are high in supplements and incorporate every one of the nutrients and minerals you want. Consolidate a scope of complete dinners, including proteins, solid fats, and veggies.

5. Restricted Protein and Carbohydrates: The FMD as a rule underlines sound fats while decreasing protein and starch consumption. This is a part of the arrangement to support fast cell and metabolic modifications.

6. Hydration: All through the FMD, keep up with sufficient hydration. To assist with hydration, take water, natural teas, and other non-caloric beverages.

7. Supplements: To ensure the utilization of crucial supplements, a few FMD regimens exhort utilizing specific enhancements. Minerals and nutrients could be remembered for these enhancements.

8. Slow Renewed introduction of Foods: Once again introduce customary meals each in turn when the FMD cycle has finished. To move once again into your customary eating regimen, begin with dinners that are high in supplements and effortlessly processed.

9. Watch out for your physical and emotional well-being: Notice the manner in which your body responds to the FMD. In the event that you experience any unfortunate results, ponder changing the system or looking for exhortation from an expert.

10. Emphasize as Necessary: For conceivable well-being benefits, certain individuals intermittently add the FMD into their routine. Yet, it's significant to change the recurrence in view of your remarkable objectives and well-being circumstances.

2.1.14 Carb Cycling with Fasting

A diet known as "Carb Cycling with Fasting" alternates days of varied carbohydrate consumption with periods of fasting. With this strategy, nutritional intake is optimized, metabolic flexibility is supported, and fat loss may be enhanced. The following is a general guide to carb cycling when fasting:

1. Establish Fasting Windows: Decide on a particular intermittent fasting strategy, such as the 16/8 technique or any other variant. The typical fasting window is between 12 and 20 hours.

2. Carbohydrate Cycle consumption: Arrange different carbohydrate consumption days. For instance, set up days of the week that are higher, moderate, and lower in carbohydrates.

3. Carbohydrate Timing: To support energy demands, aim to consume a bigger share of your carbs around your exercises on days when you consume more carbohydrates. When cutting back on carbs, try splitting up your intake more equally or concentrating on nutrient-dense, low-carb foods.

4. Select Complex carbs: Give healthy foods like fruits, vegetables, and whole grains priority when it comes to complex carbs. Steer clear of refined and highly processed carbs.

5. Protein Intake: Make sure you're getting enough protein to help with muscle growth and repair. Add sources of lean protein such as fish, chicken, tofu, and lentils.

6. Healthy Fats: For satiety and general health, include foods high in healthy fats, such as avocados, nuts, seeds, and olive oil, in your diet.

7. Hydration: Make sure you drink enough water after you eat and stay

well-hydrated during the fasting time.

8. Supplements: To make sure you satisfy your nutritional needs, especially on lower-carb days, think about supplementing with vital elements including vitamins and minerals.

9. Training Schedule: To enhance energy levels and recuperation, schedule your higher-carb days around longer, more strenuous workouts.

10. Keep an Eye on Your Physical and Mental Health: Observe how your body reacts to fasting and carb cycling. Adapt your strategy according to your state of mind, vitality, and general health.

11. Individualize Your Approach: Modify the frequency of fasting and carb cycling in accordance with your own tastes, health objectives, and reactions to the nutritional plan.

12. Consult with an expert: Get tailored advice from a certified dietitian or healthcare expert before combining carb cycling with fasting, particularly if you have underlying medical issues or special nutritional demands.

It's important to remember that different people respond differently to carb cycling combined with fasting, so this strategy might not work for everyone. Prioritize your health above everything else, and get medical advice before making any big dietary or fasting adjustments.

2.2 Building Your 21-Day Plan

2.2.1 Setting Clear Goals

Defining goals for intermittent fasting calls for a well-thought plan.

1. Define Your Objectives: Be able to justify the intention of eventually

building intermittent fasting into your everyday routine. No matter if we are speaking about weight control, enhanced energy, or anything else, the answer is that a clear purpose is needed.

2. Be Specific: For instance, instead of an indefinite objective such as "lose weight," indicate the meaningful figure that you want to shed off in these 21 days .

3. Consider Realistic Achievements: Make sure that the goals that are set are realistic and can be met within that specified period of time. The fact that targets are realistic means that the motivation of going on with the journey is maintained and frustration is avoided.

4. Prioritize Health Metrics: If health improvement is aimed at, it is necessary to designate specific variables of health, prospective values which should be measured before the revision process, such as cholesterol levels, blood pressure etc.

5. Create a Timeline: Set 21 critical goals and create mini-milestones daily to complete the goals for the 21-day period. This makes you create a path whereby every progress is not only incremental but also makes it visible and keeps directing your focus.

6. To recognize those milestones that lie outside the scale such as more energy maybe, better sleep, or better focus. Other than the scales, there are big, non-scale victories that may serve as equally important indicators of success.

7. Document Your Goals: It doesn't matter if it is in a journal, on a digital platform or even a vision board, having this enabled on a visual platform is a commitment that is so real.

8. Adjust as Needed: If your first goals seem too complicated or too simple,

feel free to change them according to your feeling and the pace of your progress in their implementation.

9. Confide in someone whether friend, family, or a support group; as to what that you want to accomplish. The notion of imposition, along with the idea of motivation can play a very important role in success of achieving the set target.

2.2.2 Crafting Personalized schedule

Making an individualized intermittent fasting program requires considering your day-to-day daily practice, inclinations, and approach to everyday life. Here is a guide to help you in making a schedule that works for you:

1. Know Your Day-to-day Routine: Look at your typical day-to-day plan, considering work, family commitments, and leisure time. Pick times when you can eat and fast that don't struggle with your timetable.

2. Select the Times for Fasting and Eating: Pick how long you need to fast and when to eat. The 16/8 procedure (16 hours of fasting, 8 hours of eating) and the 14/10 system are famous techniques. Pick a plan that works for your lifestyle.

3. Consider Normal Circadian cycles: Match your eating and fasting windows to the circadian cycles that normally happen in your body. Eating during the day and fasting during the night and night has demonstrated to find success for some individuals.

4. Bring Social Responsibilities into Account: Think about friendly exercises and social affairs. To guarantee adaptability, adjust your fasting windows to times when you could wish to have dinners with companions or family.

5. Make Consistency a Priority: Try to adhere to an everyday timetable.

Keeping up with the fast for the entire 21 days is simplified by your body being acquainted with it by means of consistency.

6. Consider Energy Levels: Monitor your degree of energy during the day. Plan your dinners for when you are generally hungry, especially assuming that you lead a functioning way of life or have requesting position plans.

7. Focus on Your Body: Know about your energy levels and indications of craving. On the off chance that you understand that a specific plan isn't appropriate for you, be versatile and make the essential changes.

8. Remain Hydrated: Try to drink enough of water during your fast. During fasting times, stay hydrated and keep up with your overall well-being by drinking water, natural teas, or other non-caloric fluids.

9. Give It A shot and Adjust: There is nobody size-fits-all way to deal with intermittent fasting. Evaluate different timetables to see one that suits you the best. While certain individuals make progress fasting at night, others like to fast in the first part of the day.

10. Seek Councel from a Professional: Talk with a certified dietitian or other medical care supplier on the off chance that you have any hidden medical problems or concerns. They can offer fitted direction as per your specific prerequisites.

It means a lot to maintain as a primary concern that the mystery is to plan a fasting plan that fits with your way of life so it very well might be supported and delighted in for longer than the 21-day plan.

2.2.3 Creating a Supportive Environment

Setting up your surroundings to assist success is part of creating a supportive atmosphere for intermittent fasting. Here is a guide to assist you in creating a nurturing environment:

1. Explain Your Plan: Tell others close to you—friends, family, or neighbors—about your intention to fast intermittently. Inform them of your schedule and ask for their cooperation and understanding.

2. Involve Your Inner Circle: If family or friends are interested in joining you for intermittent fasting, encourage them to do so. It might be more fun and inspiring to go through the procedure if you have a support network in your immediate surroundings.

3. Set Up Your Kitchen: Assemble items in your kitchen that complement your fasting regimen. Eliminate temptations that might lead to overindulgent eating during fasting. A pantry that is suitable for fasting and well-organized might be quite helpful.

4. Meal Prepping: Make meals ahead of time, especially for when others are eating. This guarantees that you always have wholesome, well-balanced meals on hand and lessens the temptation to stray from your plan.

5. Create a Dedicated Fasting Space: Choose a location where you can spend time in comfort while fasting. This can be a home office, a comfortable reading nook, or any area where you can do things other than eat.

6. Set Reminders: Make the most of technology. To help you remember when it's time to begin or stop your fast, set reminders on your calendar or phone. Reminders might assist you in staying on course, as consistency is essential.

7. Inform Your Social Circle: Explain to loved ones the advantages of intermittent fasting. This can create a more encouraging atmosphere and lessen any possible resistance or doubt.

8. Join internet Communities: Take part in social media groups or internet forums devoted to intermittent fasting. Making connections with people who share your values can offer more inspiration, guidance, and support.

9. Celebrate Success Together: Inform your network of supporters about your accomplishments and milestones. Together, you create a good atmosphere and reaffirm your commitment to fitness by celebrating tiny achievements.

Your chances of successfully implementing intermittent fasting into your lifestyle are increased when you take proactive measures to modify your surroundings and seek the help of those in your immediate environment.

2.2.4 Selecting Fasting Methods for Men and Women Over 40

For intermittent fasting to be successful and long-lasting, selecting the appropriate fasting technique is essential. This is a guide to assist you in choosing a fasting technique that works for your tastes and way of life:

1. Know several Approaches: Acquire knowledge of several intermittent fasting approaches, including the 16/8 technique, 14/10 method, 5:2 diet, and alternate-day fasting. Every technique has a different strategy for eating and fasting windows.

2. Take Daily Routine into Account: Choose a fasting technique that fits in with your daily schedule and obligations. If your schedule is stable, pick a technique that works well with your way of living.

3. Customize Your Approach: Adjust your fasting strategy to suit your

unique requirements and tastes. For instance, start your eating window later in the day if you are not an early riser.

4. Assess Energy Levels: Take note of your energy levels as the day goes on. You may choose a fasting approach that permits you to eat throughout the early hours if you are an active person.

5. Assess Your Tolerance for Hunger: Determine how much hunger you can withstand while fasting. While some approaches offer shorter windows of fasting, others entail longer periods. Select a technique based on how comfortable you are.

6. Social Considerations: Consider your social events and life in general. Select a fasting schedule that works for your social gatherings, such as dinner arrangements with friends or family.

7. Experiment and Adapt: Have an open mind to trying out various approaches. Finding the fasting strategy that feels the most sustainable and natural for you may need some trial and error.

8. Combine Techniques if Required: If a rigid approach isn't your thing, you may also mix and match different fasting strategies. For instance, you may switch up your weekly routine between the 16/8 approach and the 5:2 diet.

9. Consult a Professional: Speak with a qualified dietitian or other healthcare provider if you have any underlying medical concerns or special dietary needs. They can offer tailored guidance on selecting the most appropriate fasting technique.

10. Set Realistic Goals: Match your overall wellness objectives with your fasting strategy. If losing weight is your major goal, pick a strategy that encourages cutting calories without sacrificing nutritional balance.

Always keep in mind that the secret is to identify a sustainable fasting technique that you can use for the whole 21-day plan and beyond. Evaluate your progress on a regular basis and modify your strategy as necessary.

2.2.5 Preparation and Mental Readiness

Having the necessary supplies and mental preparation is essential for an effective experience with intermittent fasting. Here's a guide to help you get ready on the inside and out:

1. Educate Yourself: Recognize the tenets and advantages of IF. Understanding the theory behind it might increase your drive and dedication.

2. Set Clear Intentions: Clearly state why you want to include short bursts of fasting. Whether it's for better health overall, more energy, or weight control, having a specific goal makes you more committed.

3. Gradual Transition: If you're not familiar with intermittent fasting, think about making a gradual change. As your body adjusts, start with shorter fasting intervals and gradually increase them.

4. Consult an expert: If you have any underlying health issues or conditions, especially before beginning any fasting program, get advice from a licensed dietitian or healthcare expert.

5. Determine Realistic Objectives: Make attainable short- and long-term objectives. Setting reasonable expectations will improve your chances of success and help you avoid being frustrated.

6. Build a Support Network: Invite family, friends, and online groups to hear about your idea. A support network offers accountability and motivation as you go on your intermittent fasting adventure.

7. Get Ready for Obstacles: Recognize possible obstacles and devise plans to surmount them. By taking the initiative, you may overcome setbacks with fortitude.

8. Mindful Eating Practices: Make mindful food choices while you eat. To improve the entire pleasure and experience, be present and relish your food.

9. Positive Affirmations: Foster an optimistic outlook. To reaffirm your dedication and remind yourself of the goals you are pursuing, use affirmations or visualizations.

10. Create a Routine: Make sure your routine fits in with when you fast. It may be simpler to incorporate intermittent fasting into your lifestyle if you maintain consistency in your everyday routine.

11. Remain Hydrated: To stay hydrated during fasting times, drink lots of water. Drinking enough water promotes general health and helps control appetite.

12. Have Patience: Recognize that it will take some time to get used to intermittent fasting. Be kind to yourself and give your body time to acclimate.

13. Track Progress: Record your progress in a journal. Throughout the 21-day plan, record not only your physical improvements but also your emotions and experiences.

14. Celebrate Small Wins: Highlight and give thanks for little triumphs along the road. Acknowledging successes encourages positive conduct.

15. Stop on the Journey: Accept intermittent fasting as a process rather than a magic bullet for better health. Savor the procedure and the beneficial outcomes it produces.

You may make intermittent fasting more successful and gratifying by emotionally and physically preparing yourself.

2.3 Fasting Tips and Frequently Asked Questions

Here are some fasting tips to help with your intermediate fasting process. The accompanying counsel will assist you with taking full advantage of your IF experience:

1. Remain Hydrated: To stay hydrated during fasting times, drink enough water. As well as being by and large allowed, home-made teas and dark espresso (without cream or extra sugar) can likewise assist with smothering hunger.

2. Select Supplement Thick Foods: During your dinner windows, focus on eating whole, supplement thick food varieties. For a sound eating routine, give need to organic products, vegetables, lean meats, and whole grains.

3. Plan Adjusted Meals: Plan your meals ahead of time to ensure they are supple and thick. By doing this, indulging during eating times might be kept away from.

4. Pay attention to Your Body: Know about your body's signs of craving and fullness. Eating till you're fulfilled however not excessively full is significant.

5. Mindful During Meals: Take on a mindful eating style. Bite tenderly, relish each chomp, and partake in the preferences. This makes eating more agreeable all around.

6. Attempt elective Fasting Windows: If the 16/8 methodology isn't your thing, attempt a couple of other fasting windows to see which one turns out best for your preferences and lifestyle.

7. Remain Consistent: Stick to a customary fasting routine. Routineness could work with adherence to the program by helping your body in becoming acquainted with it.

8. Incorporate Actual Activity: Make ordinary time for active work in your day to day plan. Exercise can work on broad prosperity and be utilized related to intermittent fasting.

9. Make Rest a Priority: Ensure you get sufficient rest. Great rest can help upgrade your fasting experience and back up your body's normal capabilities.

10. Oversee Stress: Participate in pressure decrease exercises like yoga, profound breathing, or reflection. Stress might antagonistically affect your overall well-being as well as your ability to follow your fasting plan.

11. Break Your fast Mindfully: Begin the day with a filling and sound lunch. To ensure you get all the energy you require, including an assortment of macronutrients.

12. Remain Adaptable: Change your fasting plan depending on the situation. To keep a fair methodology, change your fasting windows because of occasions in your lifestyle or social obligations.

13. Monitor development: Archive your physical and profound changes as well as your general turn of events. You might utilize this to make any fundamental alterations.

14. Reconsider Your Goals: Survey your targets consistently and make changes considering your experience and developing conditions.

15. Look for Proficient Guidance: For individualized direction, talk with an enlisted dietitian or medical services proficient in the event that you have a particular medical problem or request..

Frequently Asked Questions About Intermittent Fasting

1. What are a few common methods for doing intermittent fasting? The 16/8 method (16 hours of fasting, 8 hours of eating), the 5:2 eating method (comprising of five days of regular eating followed by two non-sequential long stretches of calorie limitation), and alternate-day day fasting are famous methodologies.

2. Is it suitable for everybody to fast intermittently? It probably won't be proper for all individuals. Prior to starting, those with specific health issues, pregnant or nursing moms, and anybody with a background marked by dietary problems ought to talk with a medical services supplier.

3. Could I at any point have water when fasting? Indeed, it's vital to stay hydrated. By and large talking, during fasting times, one might hydrate, natural teas, and dark espresso (with next to no extra sugar or cream).

4. Might I at any point work out while on a intermittent fast? It is possible to exercise during times of fasting. While certain individuals like working out between dinner periods, others make progress with fasting works out. Focus on your body and make any changes.

5. Will intermittent fasting help in weight reduction? However results fluctuate, intermittent fasting can be a valuable weight reduction methodology. It adds to the production of a calorie deficiency and may cause fat misfortune while keeping up with strong mass.

6. What amount of time does intermittent fasting require to deliver results? Despite the fact that results shift, certain individuals might see changes in weight and energy levels in as little as half a month. Long haul benefits much of the time need ordinary responsibility, so tolerance is vital.

7. Could I at any point stick to a intermittent fasting routine and a

specific eating regimen (vegan, keto, and so on) at the equivalent time? Blending IF in with various diets is conceivable. It is versatile and may uphold numerous dietary methods of reasoning.

8. How might I break my fast? Eat an even meal that comprises of an assortment of macronutrients (carbs, fats, and proteins) to break your fast. Avoid processed or fatty dinners in abundance.

9. Could I at any point travel with a intermittent fast? Intermittent fasting is adaptable, to be sure. Consider your movement agenda while booking your fasting periods and ensure the things you pick suit your dietary patterns.

10. Does intermittent fasting have any conceivable negative effects? Beginning unfavorable impacts for certain people might incorporate cerebral pains, crabbiness, or changes in rest designs. These as often as possible disappear as the body changes. Talk with a medical care supplier in the event that you have any worries.

11. Could I at any point have tea or espresso during my fast notwithstanding water? Indeed, during times of fasting, non-caloric beverages like natural tea and dark espresso are ordinarily allowed.

12. Might intermittent fasting at any point improve fixation and mental clarity? During fasting periods, certain individuals experience expanded mental clearness and consideration. This is presumably in light of the fact that their glucose levels are consistent and their ketone age is raised.

13. Which part does autophagy play in occasional fasting? Fasting might advance the cell fix process known as autophagy. In spite of the fact that reviews are as yet being directed, it is imagined that intermittent fasting advances autophagy, which benefits cell well-being.

14. Might irregular fasting at any point upgrade insulin sensitivity? It is conceivable that IF will further develop insulin responsiveness and lower the gamble of type 2 diabetes. Look for the insight of a clinical master for custom fitted direction.

15. What is the suggested recurrence of irregular fasting? There is no set recurrence for IF. Certain individuals do it consistently, while others, contingent upon their inclinations, could pick specific days or stick to additional adaptable timetables.

16. Might IF at any point diminish inflammation? IF can offer mitigating benefits, as per some exploration. Individual responses vary, however, and further review is expected in this field.

17. Is it alright for senior to fast intermittently? For seniors, intermittent fasting can be protected, however it ought to be done cautiously. It is ideal to talk with a medical care supplier, especially in the event that there are hidden health issues.

18. What is the effect of intermittent fasting on chemicals, for example, leptin and ghrelin? Better administration of craving might result from intermittent fasting's consequences for satiety and yearning chemicals, for example, leptin and ghrelin.

Review that each individual will respond diversely to irregular fasting, so focus on your body's signs and see a specialist assuming you have a specific medical problem.

3

Chapter 3

Nutrition Essentials

3.1 Role of Macro Nutrients in IF

Polyvalent nutrients commonly referred to as macronutrients supply energy that the body needs to be in its works functionally, and such nutrients include:

1. Proteins:

Importance:

- Fundamental Building Blocks: The basic building blocks of the body are proteins, and these nutrients are very critical for the development and maintenance of the muscle tissue, connective tissues, and organs.
- Hormones and Enzymes: Proteins are regulators that act as hormones; they drive various physiological functions and as enzymes; they trigger chemical reactions.
- Immune System Support: The immune system is essential in operating, and it is because of the antibodies that are made from proteins.

Sources: Dairy products, Eggs, beef, chicken, fish, beans, nuts, seeds, tofu, and plant protein sources.

2. Fats:
Importance:

- Energy Storage: Fats act as a concentrated but efficacious reserve for storage of energy in the body.
- Cell construction: Fats are very important in the structure and function of cells. They are essential at forming parts of the cell membrane of cells.
- Hormone Production: Fats are involved in the signaling processes and the process of synthesis of hormones.

Sources: Nuts, vegetable seeds, avocado, olive oil, fish fatty, and vegetable plant oil are rich in healthy fats.

3. Carbohydrates:
Importance:

- Energy Source: The body draws its energy from carbohydrates, and this energy is easily accessible.
- Brain Function: When the human body digests carbohydrates, this gives the glucose that the brain needs to function correctly.
- Dietary Fiber: More specifically, complex carbohydrates are very important in fiber diets required for healthy digestion.

Sources: Whole grains, fruits, vegetables, legumes, and starchy vegetables are good sources of carbohydrates.

Balancing Macronutrients
1. Determine Daily Caloric Needs: Your calorie needs are determined,

considering your age, gender, activity level, and, as you mentioned, health objectives. This provides a starting point for allocating macronutrients.

2. Set Protein Intake: Calculate your protein intake, where you need to get enough grams of protein that are generally needed to maintain muscles and support recovery process. Protein is crucial during intermittent fasting to prevent muscle loss. Generally, protein intake ranges from 15-25% of total daily caloric intake.

3. Allocate Healthy Fats: Certain amount of calories that you eat every day should be directed on healthy fats. These include monounsaturated and polyunsaturated fats, found in sources like avocados, nuts, seeds, and olive oil. Fats typically make up around 20-35% of total daily caloric intake.

4. Distribute Carbohydrates: Divide the true amount of remaining calories to carbohydrates. Opt for complex carbohydrates, as they provide sustained energy and support overall health. Carbohydrates usually constitute 45-65% of total daily caloric intake.

5. Adapt Ratios to Fasting Windows: Look at your gastric ratios depending on your hours of fasting. For instance, you might focus on higher protein intake during eating windows to support muscle protein synthesis.

6. Prioritize Nutrient-Dense Foods: It should always be those nutrient-rich foods that contain necessary vitamins and minerals.This ensures you meet your micronutrient needs despite potential caloric restrictions during fasting.

7. Stay Hydrated: Your hydration levels should be well monitored because hydration also aids in digestion and the assimilation of nutrients. Water is especially important during fasting periods.

8. Include Fiber-Rich Foods: Add more fiber rich foods, and include such

foods like fruits, vegetables, beans and whole grains in the table to favor the digestive system. Fiber can contribute to a feeling of fullness, helping manage hunger during fasting.

9. Monitor Portion Sizes: For another thing, control your portion sizes to avoid being overweight or underfed. Adjust quantities based on your individual energy needs and goals.

9. Experiment and Adjust: We all have distinctive nutritional needs and are sometimes unique in our person, so do not be afraid to make experiments. Observe what happens to your body after consuming different macronutrient ratios and adjust at your own discretion.

3.2 The Role of Micronutrients in IF

1. Vitamin A: Crucial for skin well-being, immunological reaction, and visual perception.

Sources: Yams, carrots, kale, eggs, liver.

2. Vitamin C: Acts as a cancer prevention agent, supports insusceptibility, and advances the development of collagen for sound skin.

Sources: Broccoli, strawberries, chime peppers, oranges, and lemons.

3. Vitamin D: Fundamental for bone well-being, invulnerable framework control, and calcium ingestion.

Sources: Sunlight exposure, fatty fish (salmon, mackerel), fortified dairy products.

4. Vitamin E: A cancer prevention agent advances skin well-being by protecting cells from oxidative mischief.

Sources: Vegetable oils, broccoli, spinach, and nuts (almonds, sunflower seeds).

5. Vitamin K: Imperative for bone digestion, blood coagulation, and cardiovascular well-being.

Sources: Brussels fledglings, broccoli, and mixed greens (kale, spinach).

6. N-Vitamins (B1, B2, B3, B5, B6, B7, B9, and B12): They play various roles in cerebrum capability, DNA amalgamation, and energy digestion.

Sources: Vegetables, dairy items, meat, poultry, fish, and entire grains.

7. Calcium: Essential for solid bones and teeth, strong compression, and blood coagulation.

Sources: Dairy items, invigorated plant-based milk, mixed greens (kale, broccoli).

8. Iron: Crucial for blood oxygen conveyance, which turns away iron deficiency.

Sources: Fish, poultry, lentils, red meat, and sustained cereals.

9. Zinc: Advances cell digestion, wound recuperating, and immunological capability.

Sources: Nuts, seeds, meat, fish, vegetables.

10. Copper: Adds to collagen creation, iron digestion, and cancer prevention agent protection.

Sources: Organ meats, shellfish, nuts, seeds, and entire grains.

11. Selenium: Fills in as a cancer prevention agent and improves immunological reaction and thyroid capability.

Sources: Brazil nuts, salmon, chicken, and entire grains.

12. Magnesium: Indispensable for bone well-being, energy digestion, and the strength of muscles and nerves.

Sources: Entire grains, vegetables, nuts, and seeds; mixed greens.

13. Potassium: Potassium keeps up with liquid homeostasis, assists control with blooding pressure, and advances muscle and nerve capability.

Sources: Oranges, potatoes, tomatoes, beans, bananas, and potatoes.

14. Iodine: Fundamental for the combination of thyroid chemical, which advances metabolic capability.

Sources: Dairy items, fish, and iodized salt.

15. Folate (Vitamin B9): During pregnancy, fundamental for cell division, DNA union, and fetal turn of events.

Sources: Citrus organic products, mixed greens, vegetables, and sustained cereals.

16. Chromium: Advances insulin activity, which assists control with blood sugar levels.

Sources: Lean meats, nuts, broccoli, and entire grains.

17. Manganese: Advances the improvement of new bone, cell reinforcement security, and metabolic capabilities.

Sources: Mixed greens, vegetables, nuts, and entire grains.

18. Phosphorus: Fundamental for the strength of the bones and teeth, cell design, and energy digestion.

Sources: Meat, fish, dairy items, nuts, and seeds are great wellsprings of phosphorus.

Balancing Micronutrients

Adjusting micronutrients during IF is basic for meeting your body's essential prerequisites. Here are a few suggestions to assist you with keeping a reasonable admission of micronutrients during intermittent fasting.

1.Expand Your Diet: Eat different whole food varieties, including natural products, vegetables, entire grains, lean meats, and sound fats. This assortment builds the possibilities of getting a large number of micronutrients.

2. Bright Products of the soil - Eat various beautiful leafy foods. unmistakable tones regularly address particular micronutrients, and a different eating routine advances a harmony between nutrients and minerals.

3. Incorporate Lean Proteins: Center around lean protein sources such chicken, fish, beans, tofu, and low-fat dairy. Proteins offer fundamental amino acids and minerals.

4. Integrate Nuts and Seeds: Nuts and seeds are high in supplements and incorporate fundamental nutrients and minerals. Incorporate various nuts and seeds with your meals or as bites.

5. Pick Entire Grains: Select entire grains like earthy colored rice, quinoa, and entire wheat. These grains give more fiber, nutrients, and minerals than handled wheat.

6. Consider Strengthened Foods: Integrate invigorated food varieties into your eating regimen, especially in the event that you have dietary limitations. Braced food sources, for example, a few cereals or plant-based milk options, can help micronutrient utilization.

7. Pivot Protein Sources: Change your protein sources to get different micronutrients. For instance, shift back and forth between various kinds of fish, poultry, and plant-based nourishment.

8. Incorporate Dairy or Dairy substitutes: Dairy items and strengthened dairy substitutes incorporate calcium, vitamin D, and other fundamental minerals for bone well-being.

9. Eat Seafood: Incorporate seafood, for example, greasy fish like salmon, which incorporate omega-3 unsaturated fats and vitamin D.

10. Hydration with Micronutrient-Rich Beverages: Remain hydrated by drinking water, home-made tea, or other micronutrient-rich refreshments. A few home-made teas have cell reinforcements and other useful components.

11. Supplementation if Required: Assuming that you are experiencing issues satisfying your essential healthful necessities through diet alone, consider taking micronutrient supplements. In any case, prior to utilizing any enhancements, talk with a medical care expert.

12. Dinner Arranging and Tracking: Plan your meals to consolidate various supplement thick food varieties. Track your food utilization, particularly on the off chance that you're searching for and treating any potential micronutrient deficiencies.

3.3 Nutritional Consideration in Intermittent Fasting

3.3.1 How to Adapt Macronutrients Ratio

While changing macronutrient proportions for IF, midlife adults should consider their remarkable dietary prerequisites connected with maturing, digestion, and general well-being. This guide is planned considering midlife grown-ups:

1. Focus on Protein Intake: As we age, protein turns out to be progressively significant for keeping up with and fixing our muscles. For each kilogram of body weight, hold back nothing 1.6 grams of protein. Lean meats, poultry, fish, eggs, dairy items, and plant-based protein sources like tofu and beans ought to be generally included.

2. Alter Your Starch Utilization: Change your sugar admission as per your resilience and level of activity. For dependable energy, decide for complex carbs tracked down in natural products, vegetables, and entire grains. Contemplate changing the proportion as per insulin responsiveness and active work.

3. Solid Fats for Hormonal Health: Eat food varieties high in solid fats, like olive oil, avocados, almonds, and seeds. The assembling of chemicals, which turns out to be more pivotal in midlife, is upheld by these lipids.

4. Bring Supplement Timing Into Account: Space out macronutrients during taking care of windows. To help with muscle protein combination and general energy circulation, contemplate consuming some more protein promptly in the day.

5. Keep up with Hydration: Drinking sufficient water is significant, particularly as we age and our capacity to feel thirst might melt away. Add hydrating dinners like leafy foods, water, and natural teas.

6.   Calcium and Nutrient D: Ensure you are getting enough of these supplements for solid bones. Add dairy items or their braced partners, greasy fish, and daylight openness to advance the creation of vitamin D.

7.   Consolidate Omega-3 Greasy Acids: For heart and mind well-being, incorporate wellsprings of omega-3 unsaturated fats, like pecans, flaxseeds, and greasy fish (salmon, mackerel).

8.   Careful Sodium Intake: Focus on how much sodium you consume, especially in the event that you have heart issues. Pick entire, natural dinners at every possible opportunity, and utilize less high-sodium sauces.

9. Fiber-Rich Foods: To advance stomach related well-being and control glucose levels, remember food sources high for fiber, like natural products, vegetables, and entire grains.

10.   Adjust Contingent upon Individual Well-being issues: Consider a specific clinical issues or doctor prescribed drugs that can influence dietary prerequisites. Look for counsel from a certified nutritionist or medical care expert to redo macronutrient proportions to meet explicit well-being needs.

11.   Diminish Added Sugar Intake: Decrease how much added sugar consumed, since it can affect your general well-being. Select products with natural sugars instead.

12.   Normal Actual Activity: Partake in power lifting and cardiovascular activity consistently. This advances metabolic well-being overall and may affect how macronutrients are utilized.

3.3.2 Balancing Micronutrients Ratio in IF

Thinking about the exceptional nourishing prerequisites connected to growth, midlife adults should adjust their micronutrient utilization while taking part in intermittent fasting. This guide is planned in view of the process:

1. Vegetables and Natural products with Colors: Make a scope of dynamic leafy foods a need to ensure a great many cell reinforcements, minerals, and nutrients. Supplements are habitually demonstrated by unmistakable tones.

2. Verdant Greens: To get your fill of nutrients A, C, and K as well as minerals can imagine calcium and magnesium, incorporate verdant green vegetables like spinach, kale, and Swiss chard.

3. Citrus Products of the soil - Incorporate citrus foods grown from the ground for L-ascorbic acid and cell reinforcements, which help the invulnerable framework and give essential cancer prevention agents.

4. Calcium and Nutrient D: Ensure you're getting enough of these supplements for solid bones. Add dairy items or their sustained partners, greasy fish, and daylight openness to advance the creation of vitamin D.

5. Omega-3 Greasy Acids: Eat food varieties high in omega-3 unsaturated fats, like pecans, flaxseeds, and greasy fish (salmon, mackerel), for the wellbeing of your heart and mind.

6. Lean Proteins: To keep up with solid wellbeing and supply important amino acids, decide for lean protein sources like fish, chicken, tofu, and lentils.

7. Iron-Rich Foods: To upgrade oxygen transport in the blood, eat iron-rich food varieties such lean meats, lentils, and braced oats.

8. Fiber-Rich Foods: Remember food varieties high for fiber, like organic products, vegetables, and entire grains, to help solid processing and glucose control.

9. Magnesium and Potassium: To help circulatory strain the board and solid capability, remembering food sources high for magnesium (nuts, seeds, entire grains) and potassium (bananas, oranges, potatoes).

10. Hydrate with Micronutrient-Rich Drinks: Drink a lot of water and add natural teas for additional cell reinforcement security. Drink less caffeine- and sugar-filled drinks.

11. Limit Sodium Intake: To advance cardiovascular well-being, know about how much sodium you consume. Limit the use of high-sodium sauces and select whole, natural feasts.

12. Cancer prevention agent Rich Foods: To balance oxidative pressure welcomed on by , remember food sources high for cell reinforcements, like dull chocolate, green tea, and vivid vegetables.

13. B Vitamins: To support energy digestion and mental capability, eat food varieties high in B-nutrients, like entire grains, chicken, fish, and mixed greens.

14. Adapt to Explicit Well-being problems: Consider specific clinical issues or physician recommended drugs that can influence the necessities for specific micronutrients. Look for guidance from a certified nutritionist or medical care supplier to redo micronutrient utilization to meet explicit wellbeing needs.

15. Control and diversity: To ensure an equilibrium of fundamental supplements in your eating regimen, put an accentuation on control and variety. Avoid very confined slims down since they could cause dietary

lopsided characteristics.

A comprehensive and different way to deal with diet is important to adjust midlife people's utilization of micronutrients. Since every individual's requests are interesting, talking with a clinical master or qualified dietician can offer customized counsel in view of individual necessities and well-being goals.

3.4 Dealing with Hunger and Cravings

1. Hydration is Key: Make sure you drink enough amounts of water, especially during periods of not eating, such as during fasting. Adequate water aids in the ability to control body temperatures and no doubt helps curb cravings.

2. Nutrient-Dense Meals: Emphasize on keeping to balanced meals, which should be a mix of lean proteins, healthy fats, and fiber-rich foods. These two blends provide consistent energy sustainability and lower the urge to consume carbohydrates.

3. Meal Timing Flexibility: Try to adapt a less difficult intermittent fasting window to match your body better. You can choose your own peroid to eat and should tailor the experiment to one that works for you.

4. Mindful Eating: Now, pay attention to the cues of hunger or fullness. The rate of eating and enjoying every bite can help to maintain the desire and at the same time enjoying the satisfaction of having a meal.

5. Include Whole Foods: Pick whole, minimally processed food options. They contain important nutrients and may even help improve overall personal health.

6. Consider Supplements: Go into the use of supplements with a healthcare

professional, such as vitamins and minerals, for what you may gain from using them at this point life.

7. Physical Activity: Play an active life with regularly physical activity that has both aerobic and resistance capacity. You can exercise to keep their weight under check, be happier and ultimately lead better lives.

8. Prioritize Stress Reduction: Use several relaxation techniques like meditation, yoga, or any others to help you take care of stress. The high level of stress can lead to heating up and food carvings.

9. Sleep Quality: Be sure to get sufficient and good-quality sleep. Sleep deprivation can influence hunger hormones and lead to cravings and overheating.

10. Mind-Body Connection: Practice being mindful of emotional triggers for cravings. Being aware of the relationship between emotions and food can assist you in making better conscious decisions.

11. Meal Consistency: Strive for regular meal times. It stabilizes the internal clock in your body, so it can reduce cravings and overheating sensations.

12. Incorporate Variety: A variety of foods should be in your meals. This not only gives a wide range of nutrients but also makes the diet fun, which makes cravings less possible.

13. Social Support: Tell your IF story to your friends or relatives. Having a support network can make it easier to follow the plan and overcome obstacles.

14. Regular Check-ups: Regularly undergo health follow-ups and discuss on how often you practice intermittent fasting with your medical professional.

15. Educate Yourself: Be updated with the midlife dietary requirements. Knowing how your body's needs may alter helps you decide on what diet to take during intermittent fasting.

4

Chapter 4

Overcoming Challenges

4.1 Common Pitfalls in Intermittent Fasting and How to Avoid Them

What are the most typical errors made when fasting intermittently?

1. Selecting the incorrect application for your needs: There are several options for alternating patterns of fasting. It's critical to locate anything that complements your daily schedule and way of living. If not, you might not follow it well or quit up on it.

The following are the prevalent forms of intermittent fasting:

16/8: You set up an 8-hour window for eating throughout the day, and then you fast for 16 hours, generally including the night.

The 5:2 Diet involves choosing two days a week to consume 500–600 calories or less, and then eating regularly on the other days.

Alternate-Day Fasting: This involves switching off between days when you eat normally and days when you only take in 25% of your daily caloric requirements.

Eat Stop Eat: This is a once or twice-weekly 24-hour fast.

Warrior Diet: This entails having no food for 20 hours and eating every meal within 4 hours of each other.

What to do: Try out various alternatives or durations of time until you discover what works best for you.

2. You don't have smooth advances: It very well might be hard to suddenly change to eating like clockwork or without eating by any means assuming you were acquainted with eating like clockwork and in the middle between. This could cause you to feel insightful, disturbed, and uncomfortable with your eating plan.

What to do: Stretch your fasting periods judiciously to assist the change with going much more easily. You might get going with a 10- or 11-hour window and eat frequently.

3. Eating exorbitant measures of calories: Many individuals confuse the idea of this eating plan and indulge inside the designated hours since they accept they merit it or that they might eat limitless sums. Subsequent to fasting, certain individuals have solid hunger and eat exorbitant amounts of food rapidly without acknowledging it.

What to do: Since the frontal cortex requires 20 minutes to select completely, at meals, particularly the first, nibble completely and slowly. Moreover, polishing off tea or water before dinner might assist you with feeling more full faster.

4. Maintaining a very strict diet: Some people eat very little in order to lose weight as fastly as possible. Indeed, even while you will lose fat rapidly, you risk losing bone and bulk.

Moreover, you risk putting on weight fastly on the off chance that you quit your eating regimen since your body will not acquire the nutrients it needs.

Detailed instructions on how to proceed:

It's critical to move toward intermittent fasting with alert, considering your own necessities, inclinations, and well-being objectives.

5. The food varieties you are picking are not the best ones: We for the most part delude ourselves into believing that we can eat all that we need while following this eating plan. It ought to be obvious that eating handled meats and starches (like sausages), low quality food, or desserts can sabotage your endeavors to keep a solid weight and constitution.

What to do: Pick dinners that are high in strong protein, such as veggies, entire grain cereals, crude, unsalted almonds, and different natural products.

6. You don't give your body sufficient water: Water is quite possibly the most essential thing we ought to never ignore or disregard over the course of the day. Drinking much water can cause you to feel more full and lessen the probability that you will become dried out, which is particularly useful assuming you are fasting.

What to do: Try to drink a few liters of water or teas that you make yourself throughout the day, depending on your weight, the time of year, and how much vigorous work you do. Try infusing your water with bits of fruit or making herbal infusions if you find it difficult or tedious. Because of its numerous medical advantages, bone stock is a notable decision.

Due to its drying effects, always remember to sip water after finishing an espresso.

7. You drink beverages like soda: In the event that you accept that soda pops can't be a huge eating routine guilty party since they are fluids, reconsider. A few soda pops have probably the most significant carbohydrate contents and even contain "void" calories, or calories with next to no wholesome advantage.

What to do: Supplant them with smoothies, water, or teas that you develop yourself.

8. There's insufficient profound, serene rest: To keep our bodies in balance and in good health, we need to get enough sleep. It upholds the neurological framework and chemical combination. Keep in mind that our overall health should be the primary objective of any diet, and anxiety and insomnia have a significant impact on that.

What to do: Focus on rest and stress management. Try to rest for seven or nine hours consistently. Since you need to hit the sack and wake up at standard times, make an arrangement and follow it. Keep phones away to avoid distractions during sleep.

9. You surrender: Try not to blow up if, in the far-fetched occasion that you wind up surrendering each time you commit an error and conclude that this diet isn't so much for you. On the off chance that you ate unfortunate meals or at the erroneous second, it doesn't mean your endeavors were to no end.

The most ideal way to go on is to give yourself a chance to conform to this new timetable. An inordinate measure of timetable unbending nature could prompt pointless tension. Consequently, give yourself some room or investigation with an alternate sporadic fasting plan that turns out better for you.

Keep in mind: Very much contemplated feelings about irregular fasting are something similar regardless. While it may not be pragmatic for all people, it can possibly yield comparative weight reduction results as reliable dietary patterns.

4.2 Incorporating Exercise to Your IF Routine

To maximize your energy levels, try planning your exercises around the times you eat to complement your intermittent fasting. For general fitness, prioritize a combination of resistance and aerobic exercise. Drink plenty of water and break your fast with a well-balanced meal that will aid in the repair of your muscles by providing both protein and carbs. Pay attention to how your body feels during periods of fasting and modify the intensity and timing of your workouts accordingly.

Include high-intensity interval training (HIIT) to maximize metabolic gains and effective burning of calories. If you want to make exercising sustainable, pick enjoyable hobbies. Pay attention to when you consume nutrients, making sure you get enough protein to maintain and rebuild your muscles. For individualized guidance based on your health and fitness objectives, think about speaking with a healthcare provider or fitness specialist.

Moreover, give consistency precedence over intensity. Regular moderate exercise can be more maintainable than short bursts of high intensity. Try a variety of workouts to keep things fresh and avoid getting monotonous. Observe your body's cues and modify your fasting and exercise schedule as necessary.

Look into activities that fit your lifestyle, including cycling, walking, or working out at home. Include strength exercise to increase fat reduction and metabolism. Remain aware of how your body reacts to exercise and fasting, and be adaptable in modifying your regimen as necessary. To prevent burnout, gradually increase the length and intensity of your workouts. Achieving a successful incorporation of exercise into your intermittent fasting regimen requires consistency, variation, and adaptability.

To increase mobility and lower your risk of injury, think about combining stretches or yoga into your routine. To stay motivated, keep track of your progress using measurements, a notebook, or fitness apps. Drink enough water to aid in performance and recuperation during fasting and exercise. Keep in mind that every person is different, so adjust your strategy according to how your body responds to the combined fasting and exercise program. Finally, get individualized advice from a healthcare provider or fitness specialist depending on your current state of health and desired level of fitness.

As you proceed, keep an eye out for any indications of excessive weariness or overtraining. Permit sporadic days of relaxation to aid in recuperation. Try varying the time of your workouts and fasts to see what best fits your body's natural rhythm. Concentrate on creating a regimen that fits your lifestyle and is long-lasting. Keep up your nutrition knowledge to make sure your body gets the nutrients it needs to sustain activity and fasting. As you progressively enhance your intermittent fasting and exercise combination, consistency and patience are essential. In order to control stress, which can affect the results of both fasting and exercise, think about implementing mindfulness techniques like meditation or deep breathing exercises. Be mindful of your mental health and how it affects your entire quest for fitness and wellness. To keep things interesting and difficult, periodically review your objectives and modify your schedule. To improve responsibility and motivation, surround oneself with a positive and encouraging group of people or a workout buddy. Accept the path as a comprehensive strategy for well-being that takes into account both your bodily and mental well-being.To keep things fresh and avoid monotony, mix up your exercises by doing new activities like swimming, hiking, or group courses. To benefit from the natural environment and fresh air, try outdoor activities. A trained dietitian or nutritionist may offer advice on how to ensure that your diet and exercise regimen work together to provide you with the nutrients you need for long-lasting energy and recuperation. Pay attention to your body's cues and adjust your workout and fasting schedule accordingly to find a healthy balance that suits your needs.

Prioritize proper sleep hygiene as you advance to maximize your recuperation. Make your space conducive to rest, and try to get 7 to 9 hours of good sleep per night. To maintain your energy levels, break your fast with nutrient-dense foods and pay attention to your body's hunger cues. Maintain consistency in your routine since long-lasting habits are those that are created over time. To keep yourself inspired to continue your adventure of intermittent fasting and exercise, acknowledge and appreciate your minor victories. Recall that it's a slow process, and the secret to long-term success is figuring out a regimen that fits your lifestyle.

To sum up, adding exercise to intermittent fasting can be a very effective way to improve general health and well-being. Pay attention to a well-rounded strategy that incorporates different workouts, drinking enough of water, and modifying your regimen in response to your body's reactions. Consistency is key, pay attention to your body, and don't undervalue the need of getting enough sleep. Customize your plan to meet your unique tastes and way of life for a fun and long-lasting fitness journey. For individualized guidance based on your unique requirements and objectives, always seek the advice of medical or fitness specialists.

4.3 Intermittent Fasting for Midlife Men in 21 Day

4.3.1 Week 1

Day 1: Adaptation Phase
Morning: Start the day with a herbal tea or a glass of water. This aids in reviving dehydration.

Midday: Break your fast with a well-balanced meal, including whole-grain bread and scrambled eggs with spinach.

Afternoon: Drink water or herbal tea to stay hydrated. Choose a snack like a handful of almonds or a piece of fruit if you're hungry in between meals.

Evening: Savor grilled chicken, quinoa, and roasted veggies for a satisfying supper. After supper, begin your fasting window with the goal of waiting 16 hours until your next meal.

Day 2

Morning: Proceed with herbal tea, black coffee, or water. Continue drinking water in the morning.

Midday: Enjoy a nutrient-dense meal that includes grilled salmon, mixed green salad, and an assortment of vibrant veggies.

Afternoon: Drink lots of water. If you feel like it, pack a snack, such Greek yogurt and berries.

Evening: Steamed broccoli, sweet potatoes, and lean protein (lean beef or tofu) might be the dinner fare. After supper, start your fast.

Day 3

Morning: As on earlier days, pay attention to your morning hydration.

Midday: Choose a high-fiber, high-protein lunch, such as a whole-grain tortilla wrapped around turkey and avocado.

Afternoon: Stay hydrated and think about having a little, high-protein snack, such as cottage cheese and pineapple.

Evening: Supper may include sautéed lush greens, quinoa, and grilled fish.

After supper, start the fasting window.

Day 4

Fasting Window: Adhere to the 16-hour window for fasting. Continue starting at 8 PM on Day 1 if you started at that time.

Meal Composition: Keep putting an emphasis on whole foods by combining complex carbohydrates (quinoa, sweet potatoes), healthy fats (olive oil, almonds), and proteins (chicken, legumes).

Snacking: Remind yourself not to overindulge in snacks. If you need a snack, go for nutrient-dense options like sliced vegetables with hummus.

Hydration: Throughout the day, especially when fasting, continuously consume water.

Day 5

Meal Timing: Stay inside the 8-hour window with a regular eating schedule. For example, strive to finish your last meal by 8 PM if you break your fast at 12 PM.

Portion Control: To prevent overindulging, pay attention to portion proportions. Pay attention to the caliber of the food you eat.

Meal diversity: To guarantee a wide range of nutrients, introduce a diversity of foods.

Hydration Habits: Drink enough water, particularly during the window for fasting. For more taste, think of infused water or herbal teas.

Day 6

Meal Prepping: To make it simpler to adhere to your eating window and guarantee you have wholesome alternatives accessible, think about cooking meals in advance.

Fluid Intake: Drink electrolyte-rich drinks in addition to water to help hydrate, particularly if you exercise moderately.

Mindful Eating: Recognize your body's signals of hunger and fullness. To increase enjoyment, savor your food and eat leisurely.

Day 7

Social Considerations: Let others know when you're eating to reduce temptations and encourage you to stick to your diet.

Stress Management: To enhance general wellbeing, include stress-relieving practices like deep breathing, meditation, or gentle stretching.

Individual replies can be used to make adjustments. Always pay attention to your body's signals, and seek the guidance of a healthcare provider if necessary.

4.3.2 Week 2

Day 8

Fasting Window: If you do not feel comfortable with a 16:8 ratio, stick with an 18-hour timeframe.

Meal Composition: Mix and match complex carbohydrates (quinoa, sweet potatoes) and healthy fats (olive oil, avocado) with a range of protein sources (fish, lean meat).

Stay Hydrated: Drink lots of water throughout the fasting period and consider consuming herbal teas.

Day 9

Diversity of Meals: Experiment with other types of protein, such as plant-based sources like tofu or beans.

Interruption Fasting Techniques: If you want even more diversity, you might want to try the 5:2 method or alternate-day fasting.

Day 10

When to Eat: Be mindful of when you eat inside the designated window. A healthy breakfast is a smart way to begin the day.

Workout Schedule: Continue doing weight training and cardiovascular exercises (jogging, brisk walking) to maintain overall health.

Strategies for Hydration: It is crucial to maintain proper hydration when engaging in more intense physical exercise.

Day 11

Meal Timing: See whether you can sustain your energy levels throughout the day by consuming a larger breakfast.

Exercise Variation: Try including a variety of exercises to keep your program interesting and your body challenged.

Hydration Focus: Make sure to stay hydrated, especially before, during, and after physical activity.

Day 12

Meal Timing: Continue experimenting with the time of day you eat, and if a heartier dinner tempts you, consider having one.

Workout Routine: Try a variety of routines and incorporate activities you enjoy to keep motivated.

Hydration Habits: To stay properly hydrated, prioritize drinking lots of water along with herbal teas and high-water meals.

Day 13

Consistency: When choosing the fasting window and meal type, adhere to the planned schedule.

Workout Routine: Continue your regimen by mixing aerobic and strength training. Consider working out in a demanding manner.

Hydration: Make sure to drink lots of water throughout the day, as well as herbal teas and foods that are high in water content.

Day 14

Consistency: Maintain a regular fasting window and a balanced diet.

Reflection: Examine your body's response to the adjustments made in Week 2. Note whether your appetite, energy, or overall well-being changes at all.

Suggest: If you have any concerns or questions, consider consulting a healthcare physician to ensure that the plan aligns with your health goals.

General Recommendations for Days 13 and 14:

Meal Variety:* Make sure that your proteins, healthy fats, and complex carbohydrates are all in balance and keep your meals nutrient-dense by combining a variety of foods.

Sleep: Prioritize good sleep hygiene in order to support overall wellness.

Stress Management: To improve mental and physical health, incorporate techniques for reducing stress, such as gentle stretches or deep breathing.

As always, adjust based on your own preferences and responses. While consistency is important, you should also be aware of your body and adjust the plan as needed.

4.3.3 Week 3

Days 15–17

Fasting Window: Depending on how comfortable you are, stick to the 16:8 or 18-hour fasting window.

Meal Composition: Experiment with different protein sources, colorful veggies, and healthy fats like nuts or avocados to fine-tune nutritional ratios.

Physical Activity: Continue to combine strength and aerobic training. Evaluate your energy and change the amount of intensity as necessary.

Day 18

Fasting Strategies: To add even more variation, try more sophisticated methods like a day of OMAD (One Meal a Day).

Meal Timing: Try different times for your meals to see what gives you the most energy and satiety.

Physical Activity: Keep up your current exercise regimen, making any necessary modifications in response to your body's reaction.

Days 19–21

Meal time: Continue experimenting with the time of your meals and see how it impacts your general wellbeing.

Reflect and Adapt: Give the entire 21-day trip some thought. Examine the elements of the routine that were effective and think about making changes for long-term sustainability.

Celebration: During the 21-day period, recognize and honor the beneficial adjustments you've made to your lifestyle.

Overall Advice

Hydration: Keep drinking water and herbal teas as your main source of hydration.

Sleep and Stress Management: For general wellbeing, practice excellent sleep hygiene and engage in stress-relieving activities.

Adjust the regimen to suit your own needs and tastes. These last few days are your chance to perfect your strategy and lay the groundwork for long-lasting routines that go beyond the 21-day window.

4.4 IF Routine for Midlife Women in 21 Day

4.4.1 Week

Day 1-3 of the Adaptation Phase

Fasting Window: First of all, allot a window of 14 to 16 hours. If you have dinner at 8 PM, for instance, begin your eating window at 10 AM and finish it at 12 PM a day after.

Meal Composition: Prefer meals that are balanced in protein, healthy fats and complex carbohydrates like fish, chicken and tofu, almonds, avocado, and vegetables, whole grains.

Hydration: Drink water, herb teas, black coffee to be able to stay hydrated as this supports adaptability during the fasting period.

Snacking: In case you get hungry before the next meal, try eating some healthy snacks such as almonds, yogurt or fruits.

Day 4

Fasting Window: The adherence to a fasting window of 14 – 16 hours is standardized.

Meal Timing: Order your meals in a way that you have them within an eight hours window. Think about having a big lunch, a nutritious breakfast, and a balanced diet.

Exercise: Add mild to intense exercises which may include yoga, light weight training or a walk lasting thirty minutes.

Hydration: All day long, emphasize staying hydrated by drinking water, herbal teas are also good.

Days 5-7

Fasting Window: Maintain the 14–16 hour fasting window.

Meal Timing: Follow the 8-hour feeding window and take nutritionally rich foods in the breakfast, lunch, as well as dinner.

Exercise: Keep performing workouts at a moderate stimulus, differentiating it to some aspects in order to keep it fascinating.

Hydration: To remain hydrated, have plenty of water, herbal teas, or water with infusions.

Modifications for Women:

Hormonal Factors to Consider: Recognize that hormones change during the menstrual cycle. During different periods, modify meal plans or fasting lengths according to your energy and comfort levels.

Nutrient Intake: Make sure meals contain the necessary nutrients, taking into account the ratio of macro-to micronutrients for proper hormonal balance.

Pay Attention to Your Body: Observe your body's reaction to the fast. Adjust the fasting schedule if you feel fatigued, if your menstrual cycle is erratic, or if you have other concerns.Always adjust the routine to your unique answers, and for individualized guidance, speak with a certified dietitian or other healthcare provider.

4.4.2 Week 2

Day 8

Fasting Window: If you find it comfortable, keep to a 16:8 fasting window; if not, consider maintaining an 18-hour window.

Meal Composition: Place a focus on complex carbs (vegetables, whole grains), healthy fats (avocado, nuts), and a variety of proteins (fish, poultry, and plant-based alternatives).

Intermittent Fasting Techniques: If you're interested, experiment with various strategies like the 5:2 strategy or alternate-day fasting.

Day 9

Meal Variety: Try a variety of protein sources, including plant-based sources like beans or tofu.

Intermittent Fasting Techniques: To add variation, keep looking at various strategies like the 5:2 technique or alternate-day fasting.

Day 10

Fasting Window: Adhere to the window of choice for fasting. Observe how your body adjusts to the more sophisticated regimen.

Meal Timing: Pay close attention to when you eat inside the 8-hour window. Think about having a healthy breakfast to start the day.

Hydration Strategies: If you're doing more strenuous activity, it's important to stay hydrated.

Day 11

Meal Timing: Try having a bigger breakfast to see whether you can maintain your energy levels all day.

Exercise Variation: To keep your body challenged and interest level up, try introducing various types of exercise.

Hydration Focus: Drink enough water, especially before, during, and after exercise.

Day 12

Fasting Window:* Stick to the selected fasting window, if it seems more comfortable, using an 18-hour approach.

Meal Timing: Try different times for your meals; if a bigger dinner works for you, consider having one.

Workout Routine: To stay motivated, experiment with different routines and include things you love.

Hydration Habits: To be well-hydrated, emphasize a combination of water, herbal teas, and meals high in water.

Days 13-14

Consistency: Adhere to the prescribed schedule, making sure that meals, exercise, and fasting periods are all consistent.

Introspection: Consider how your body reacts to the modifications made in Week.

Consultation: For individualized counsel and direction, seek the assistance of a healthcare provider if necessary.

Never forget to modify the regimen in accordance with your unique tastes and reactions. These thorough analyses serve as a daily guide, but pay attention to your body's signals and modify as necessary.

4.4.3 Week 3

Day 15-17: Optimization Phase
Fasting Window: If this is comfortable then continue the 18-hour period or just stick to 16:8.

Meal Composition: Adjust ratios of nutrients to individual tastes. Adding colorful vegetables as well as different types of proteins (chicken, fish, something plant-based) and healthy fats (avocado, nuts) in every meal is worth considering.

Physical Activity: Engage in a combination of aerobic activities such as brisk walking and cycling as well strength training. Tailor the strength based on energy levels as well as preferences.

Hydration Strategies: Highlight hydration with water and herbal teas especially on fasting.

Day 18
Fasting Strategies: Introduce some new methods like a day of OMAD (One Meal a Day), to diversify.

Meal Timing: Vary meal times to see what gives sustained energy and satiation. Think about a meal rich in nutrients after the fasting window.

Physical Activity: Maintain the current regimen of exercise, adapting to the energy levels.

Day 19-21: Finalization and Reflection

Fasting Strategies: Alternatively, begin with advanced fasting methods if that is your will.

Meal Timing: Continue trying different timing for meals and note how this impacts your energy levels as well as the hunger cues. Think of a combination of proteins, good fats, and carbohydrates.

Reflect and Adapt: Spend sometime looking back at the whole 21-day trip. Evaluate which parts of the routine were successful and think about modifications for the long-term sustainability.

Celebration: Praise yourself for the healthy lifestyle changes you've introduced within the 21 days established.

Modifications for Women

Recognize the changes in hormones that occur during the menstrual cycle. During different periods, modify meal plans or fasting lengths according to your energy and comfort levels.

For hormonal balance, adjust nutrient ratios with an emphasis on colorful veggies, a variety of proteins, and healthy fats. Observe how your body reacts to more complex tactics. Think about changing the plan if you feel exhausted, notice changes in your menstrual cycle, or have other concerns. Recall that everyone reacts differently, therefore it's important to put your health first. Prior to making big dietary or activity changes, always get advice from a medical practitioner or a qualified dietician, especially if you're a reproductive age.

5

Chapter 5

Healthy and Nutritious Recipes to Aid your IF Journey

5.1 Breakfast Meal Plans for IF

5.1.1 Baked Banana Porridge

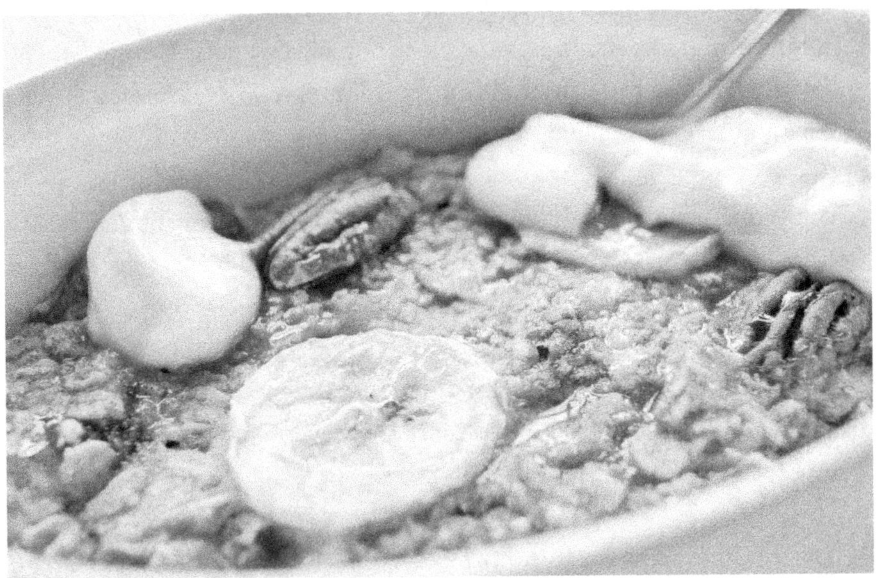

Ingredients:

- 1 cup rolled oats
- 2 ripe bananas, mashed
- 2 cups milk (or a dairy-free alternative)
- Pinch of salt
- Dash of cinnamon
- Optional toppings: nuts, honey, or sliced fresh fruits

Instructions:

1. Preheat Oven: To guarantee that the porridge bakes uniformly, preheat the oven is necessary. Preheat the oven to 350°F (175°C). Once the temperature reaches that point, put the dish inside.

2. Prepare Baking Dish: Greasing the baking dish helps to keep the porridge from sticking, which facilitates serving and cleanup. For greasing, you can use cooking spray, butter, or oil.

3. Combine Ingredients: In this stage, the porridge's essential ingredients—rolled oats, mashed bananas, milk, salt, and cinnamon—are combined. Ripe bananas naturally provide taste and sweetness.

4. Mix Well: In order to obtain a homogenous mixture, thoroughly whisk the components. Make sure the mashed bananas and milk are combined equally with the rolled oats to form a cohesive mixture.

5. Transfer to Baking Dish: Evenly distribute the mixture into the baking dish that has been buttered. This guarantees even baking and a constant texture for the whole oatmeal.

6. Bake: Baking duration is important. As the porridge bakes for 25 to 30 minutes, keep an eye on it. Achieving a golden top and a certain uniformity is the aim. In this stage, the flavors can combine and the oats can absorb the liquid.

7. Serve: Allow the porridge to cool for a few minutes after baking before cutting into portions. The dish can set even further during this brief resting period.

8. Optional Toppings: Garnish your baked banana porridge to make it uniquely yours. Crunch comes from nuts, sweetness from honey, and freshness from cut fruit. These garnishes improve the dish's taste and texture.

9. Savor: At last, indulge in the cozy baked banana porridge. This meal delivers a delicious blend of flavors and textures, perfect for breakfast or as a snack.

Please feel free to adjust the recipe to suit your tastes. For even more flavor depth, you may also think about adding other spices like nutmeg or vanilla essence. Savor the baked banana porridge you cooked yourself!

5.1.2 Chia Seed Pudding

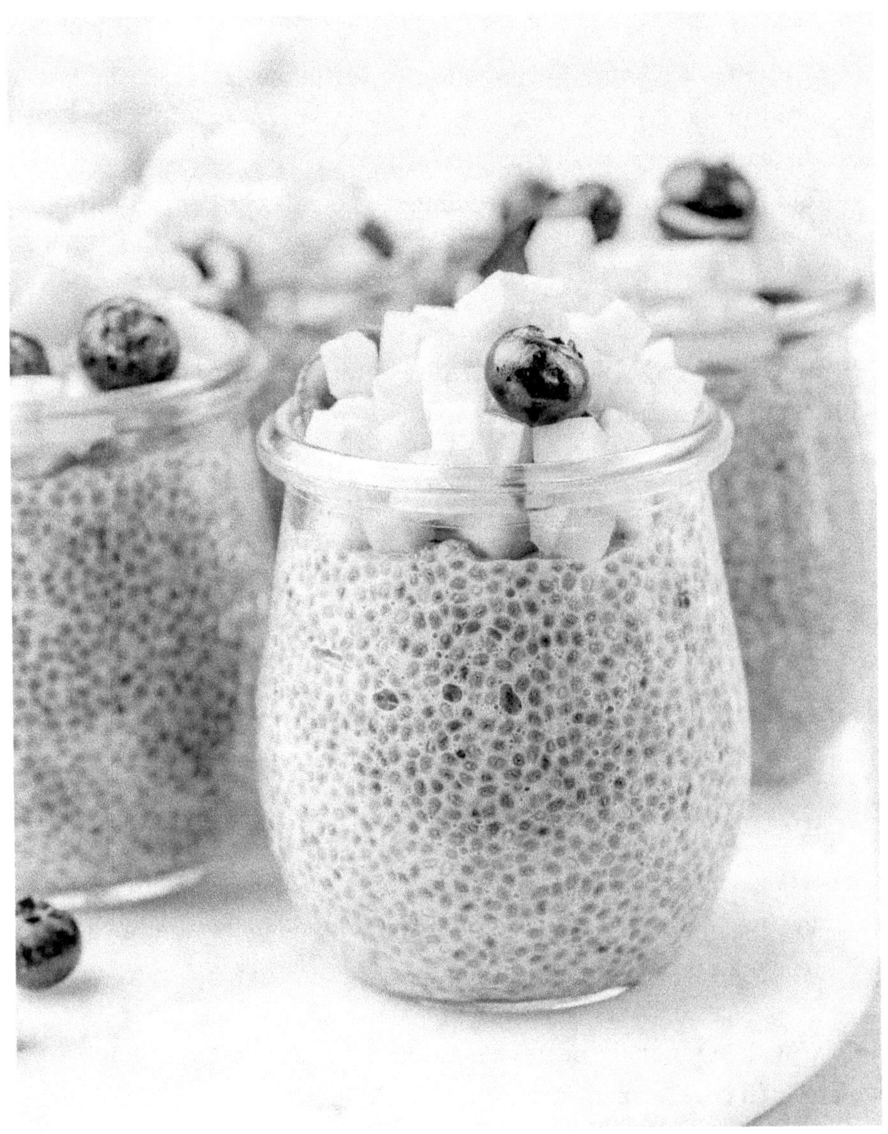

Ingredients:

- 1/4 cup chia seeds
- A cup of milk – vegan or otherwise.
- Sweetener is about a teaspoon to two teaspoons (agave syrup, maple syrup, or honey)
- 1/2 teaspoon (optional) vanilla extract
- Your favorites in toppings including the granola, nuts or fresh fruits

Instructions:

1. Chia Seeds and Milk: In a container or dish mix 1/4 cup of chia seeds with 1 cup of milk. Ensure that the chia seeds are well spread throughout by stirring it.

2. Add Vanilla Extract and Sweetener: You can add one to two teaspoons of your preferred sweetener to taste. You can modify the sweetness as you wish. You can also add 1/2 teaspoon of vanilla essence for taste.

3. Stir Thoroughly: In order to prevent clumping, thoroughly stir the chia seed mixture. Make sure the sweetener has been blended with the mixture.

4. Refrigerate: Place the jar or bowl in the fridge and cover it. After making the chia seed pudding, allow it to sit for up to three hours or better, leave it to sit overnight. The chia seeds will absorb the liquid in this time giving this mixture a pudding consistency.

5. Stir Again (Optional): Beat the pudding vigorously to prevent lumping which could have formed during the first chilling process. This procedure ensures smooth surface.

6. Add Toppings: After that, sprinkle your chosen toppings over the chia seed pudding before taking it out. You can opt to have more sugar, granola,

nuts, or fresh fruits to enhance the taste and texture.

7. Savor: Time to enjoy your chia seed pudding. You can either eat it off the jar or spoon it into a bowl.

5.1.3 Easy Veggie Omelet

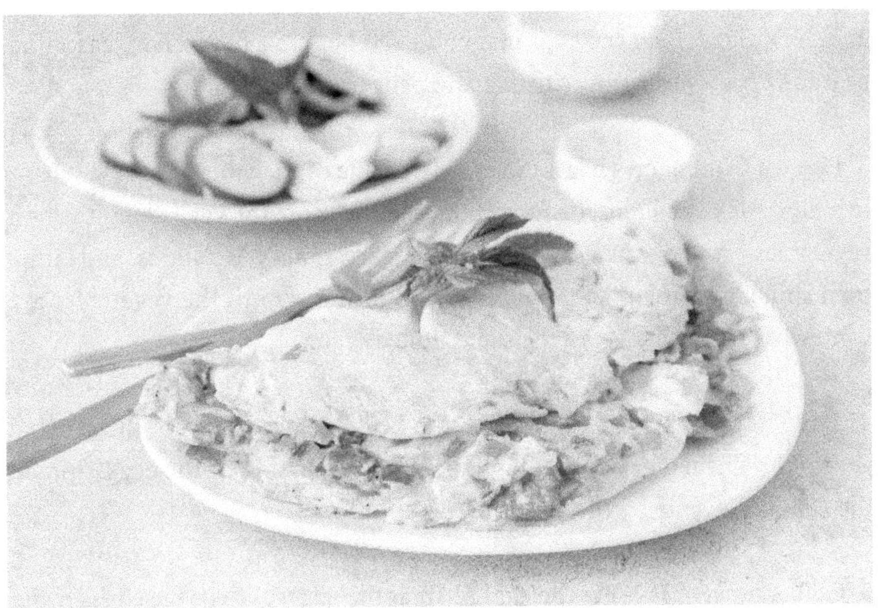

Ingredients

- 2-3 eggs
- 1/4 cup diced bell peppers (any color)
- 1/4 cup diced tomatoes
- 1/4 cup diced onions
- 1/4 cup chopped spinach or kale
- Salt and pepper to taste
- 1 tablespoon oil or butter for cooking

• Optional: grated cheese for topping

instructions

1. Onions, bell peppers, and tomatoes should be chopped. Cleave spinach or kale. These veggies will add tone, flavor, and supplements to your omelet.

2. Whisk Eggs: Beat the eggs in a bowl and beat to a foam. For seasoning, beat the eggs and season with salt and pepper.

3. Preheat Container: Heat 1 tablespoon of one or the other oil or margarine in a non-stick skillet on medium intensity and sauté the vegetables; the best vegetables for this stew are diced bell peppers, tomatoes, onions, and either torn spinach or torn kale. Sauté for 2-3 minutes until the vegetables are somewhat mellowed yet at the same time dynamic.

4. Pour Eggs Over Vegetables: Put the beaten eggs on top of the sautéed vegetables ensuring that there is a uniform dispersion of the eggs. Spread the eggs out evenly by tilting the pan.

5. Cook and Overlay: Let the eggs to sit at the edges. When the edges begin to lift, utilize a spatula to tenderly lift and crease one side of the omelet over the other, making a half-moon shape.

6. Discretionary Cheddar Besting: If you want, you can eat cheese. To allow the cheese to melt, cover the pan for a minute.

7. Complete the process of Cooking: Continue cooking for another 1-2 minutes, or until the eggs are fully set but still have a tender center. Be mindful not to overcook, as this can bring about a dry omelet. Serve: Move the veggie omelet to a plate. Decorate with extra salt, pepper, or spices whenever wanted. Enjoy: Your vegetable-filled omelet is now complete and

delicious.

8. Serve it as a morning meal thing, early lunch reason or you can serve it as a speedy and quality feast.

5.1.4 Cottage Cheese with Fruit Bowl

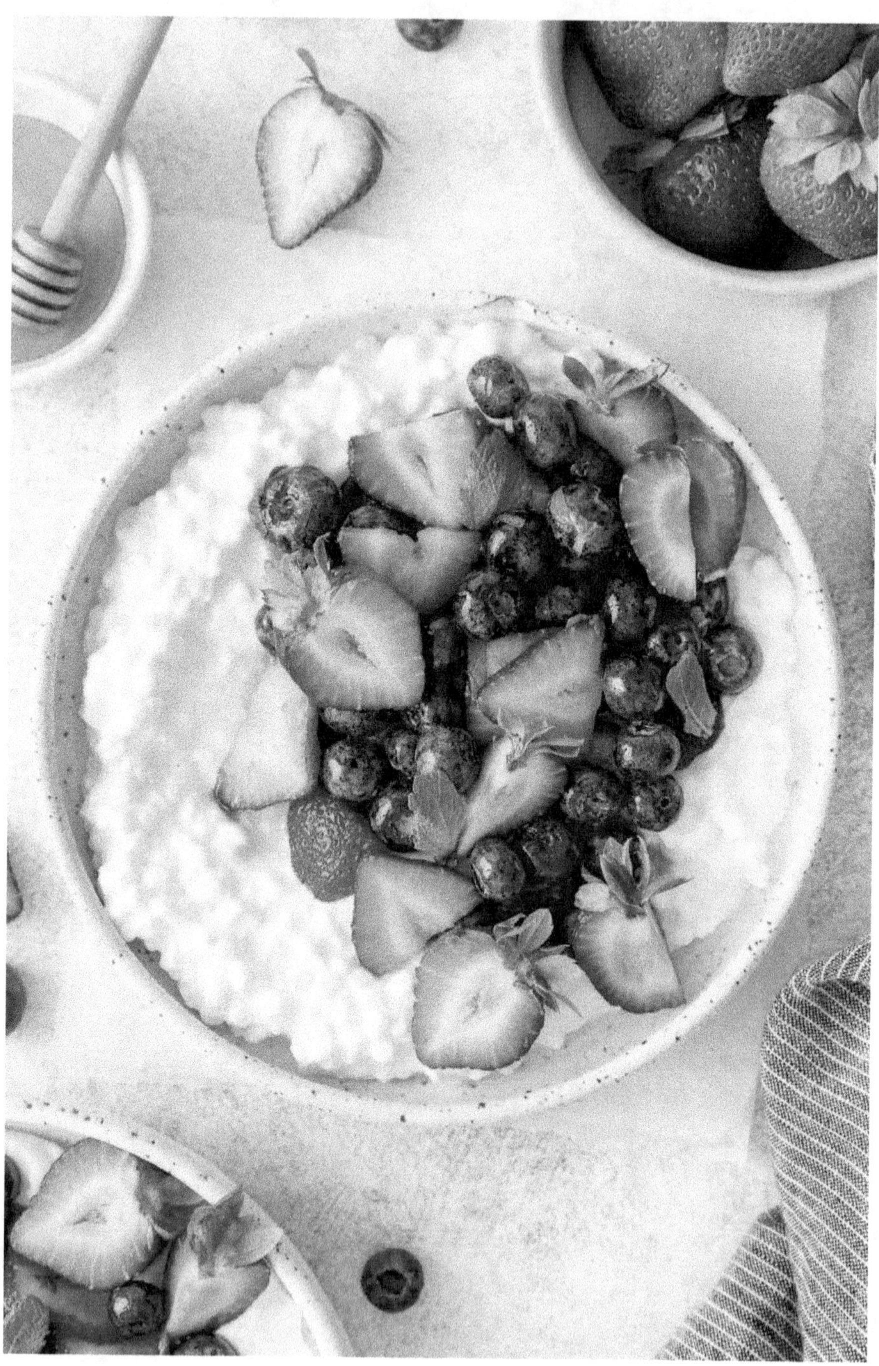

Ingredients:

- 1 cup cottage cheese
- 1 cup mixed fresh fruits (e.g., berries, kiwi, pineapple, or any of your favorites)
- 1 tablespoon honey or maple syrup (optional for sweetness)
- 1/4 cup chopped nuts (such as almonds, walnuts, or pistachios)
- Optional for crunch

Instructions:

1. Get the new natural items ready: Cut some fresh fruits into tiny pieces by washing and dicing them. Try combining various types and surfaces to create a vibrant and tasty dish of natural products.

2. Mixing Berries with Cottage Cheese: Combine with a cup of curds in a bowl. Sprinkle a fresh natural product over the curds. Optional maple syrup or honey drizzle: If you feel like adding a little sweetness, drizzle one table spoon of honey or maple syrup over the curds and strawberries. Please adjust the sweetness to your taste.

3. Not required: Add 1/4 cup chopped nuts to the top of your fruit and cottage cheese dish to improve its flavor and texture. This tactic gives it an amazing smash.

4. Stack or toss gently: To create a visually appealing meal, you may gently mix the ingredients together or stack the natural goods on top of the curds.

5. Serve: Your cottage cheese and fruit dish is best served immediately for a wholesome breakfast or snack.

6. Enjoy yourself: Smell the blend of creamy curds, crunchy almonds, and sweet natural goods. This recipe is not only incredibly tasty, but it also has a balanced protein, nutrient, and fat profile.

5.1.5 Greek Yogurt Parfait

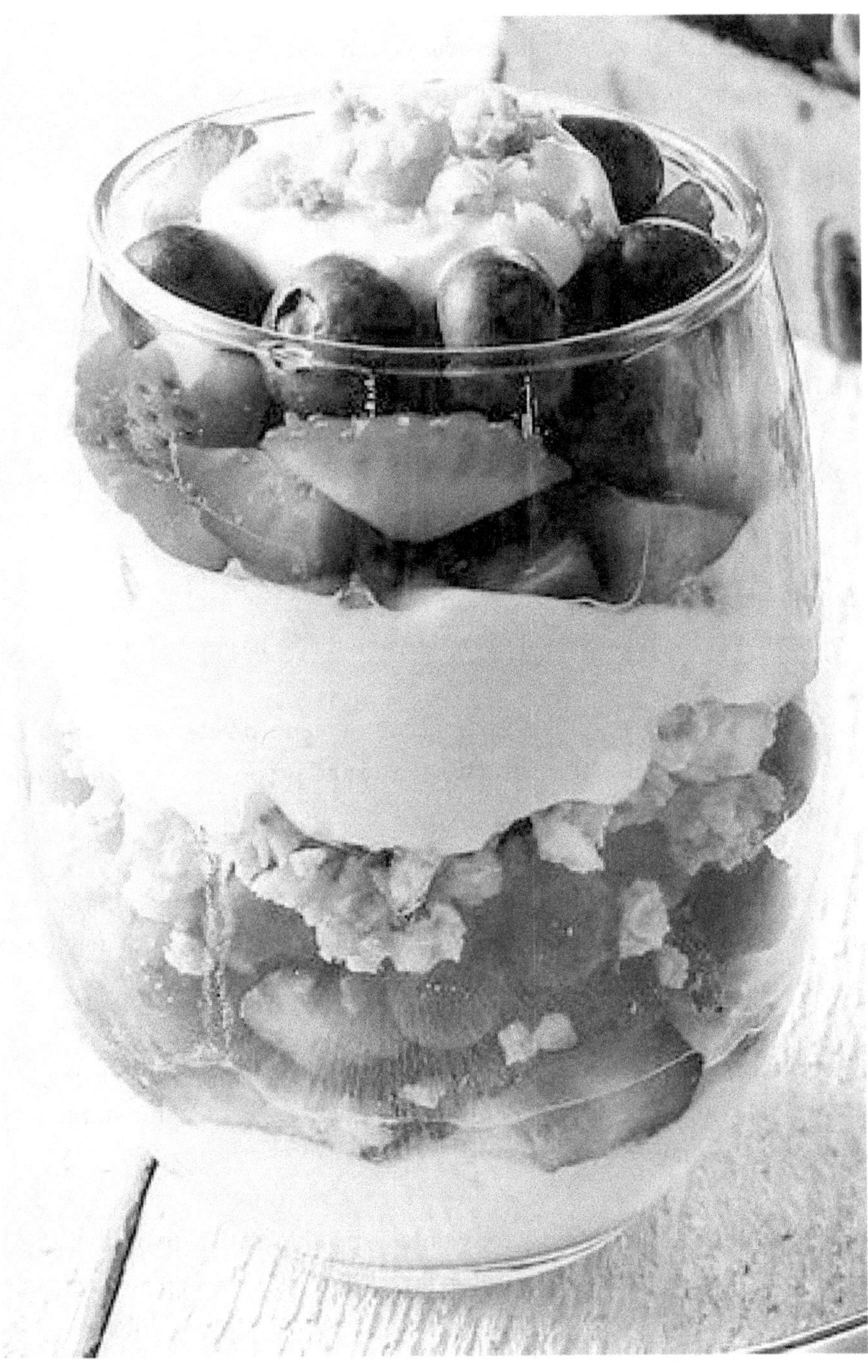

Ingredients

- A cup of Greek yogurt, either plain or enhanced
- A half cup of blended new berries, including strawberries, blueberries, and raspberries
- A half cup of granola
- 1 tablespoon of optional nuts (almonds or walnuts)
- 1 spoonful of honey or maple syrup are all you need

Instructions:

1. Greek Yogurt Layer: Line a glass or plate base with a layer of Greek yogurt. This rich, high-protein base is possible because of its creamy consistency.

2. Add Granola Layer: Sprinkle some granola on top of the Greek yogurt. The parfait gets a nice crunch from this, and it also has more fiber.

3. Top with New Berries: Dissipate a layer of blended new berries over the granola. Berries have a normally sweet taste and proposition an eruption of flavor.

4. Rehash Layers: Continue to add Greek yogurt, granola, and new berries until the glass or dish is filled. This delivers a parfait that is both delightful and outwardly engaging.

5. Sprinkle with Honey or Maple Syrup: Sprinkle 1 tablespoon of honey or maple syrup on top of the parfait to make it better. Change the sum to suit your own inclinations.

6. Discretionary Nuts: Whenever wanted, sprinkle 1 tablespoon of hacked nuts, like pecans or almonds, over top for additional surface and nutty flavor.

7. Serve Immediately: The Greek yogurt parfait makes a great breakfast, snack, or dessert because it's so fast to serve.

8. Savor: Bite on the layers of tasty berries, fresh granola, and smooth yogurt with each spoonful. This parfait isn't just delightful yet in addition a fabulous portion of fiber, protein, and cell reinforcements.

You are free to alter the parfait by incorporating your preferred toppings, nuts, or fruits. This recipe can be easily modified to suit your preferences.

5.1.6 Bone Broth Breakfast

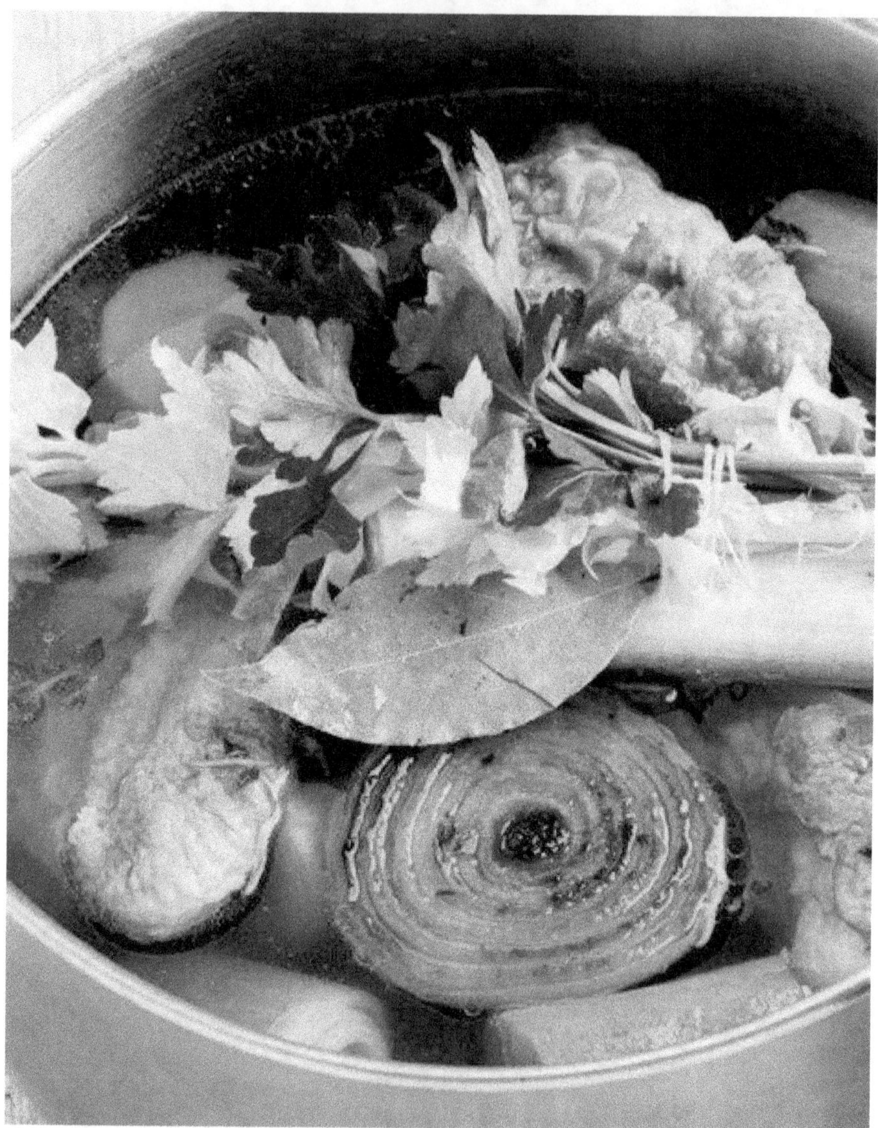

Ingredients:

- A few pounds of bones from hamburger or chicken
- One quartered onion
- 2 cut carrots
- 3 stalks of chopped celery

- Four cloves of crushed garlic
- 2 teaspoons of apple cider vinegar
- Salt and pepper
- Optional fresh herbs like rosemary or thyme; and water.

Instructions:

1. Set the oven temperature to 400°F, or 200°C. To work on the flavor, put the bones on a baking skillet and dish for around 30 minutes.

2. Put the simmered bones, celery, carrots, onion, garlic, and apple juice vinegar in a major pan.

3. Add sufficient water to the pan to cover the items. If utilizing, season with salt, pepper, and new spices.

4. Reduce the heat after bringing the mixture to a boil. For chicken bones, stew covered for no less than 4 hours, or for hamburger bones, for 8 to 24 hours. The taste gets more extravagant the more it stews.

5. Skim off any foam or particles that once in a while ascend to the top.

6. To dispose of the particles, channel the stock utilizing cheesecloth or a fine-network strainer. Subsequent to allowing it to cool, refrigerate. It will become simpler to eliminate the fat after it cements on top.

7. On the off chance that you really want it for breakfast, warm a portion of the stock.

Enjoy the bone broth's nutrients!

5.1.7 Tofu Scramble with Veggies

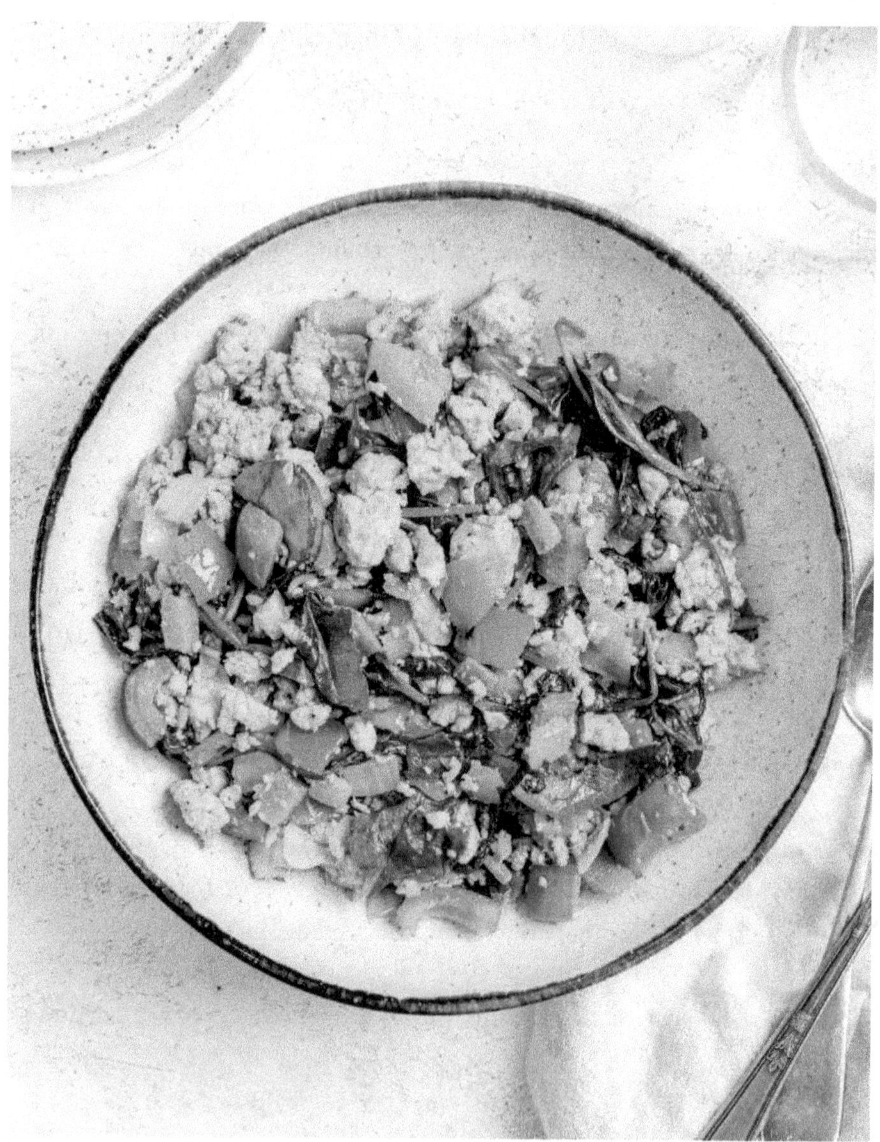

Ingredients:

- 1 block of firm tofu, pressed and crumbled.
- 1 tablespoon olive oil
- 1 small onion, finely chopped
- 2 cloves garlic, minced
- 1 bell pepper, diced
- 1 cup cherry tomatoes, halved
- 2 cups spinach or kale, roughly chopped
- 1 teaspoon of turmeric powder as a colouring agent.
- 1/2 teaspoon cumin
- Salt and pepper to taste
- Optional toppings: avocado slices, salsa, nutritional yeast

Instructions:

1. In a large skillet, heat olive oil over medium heat. Add the cut onions and garlic, fry until tender.

2. Then add diced bell pepper and fry until tender for a few minutes.

3. Add to the skillet broken tofu. Sprinkle turmeric powder, cumin to the tofu for color and taste.

4. Mix the tofu in with the turmeric adding evenly in its distribution coating the tofu.

5. Throw in cherry tomatoes and chopped spinach or kale in the skillet. Cook the vegetable until tender and while tofu absorbs the flavors.

6. Sprinkle it with salt and black pepper as preferred. Adjust the seasonings if needed.

7. Serve the tofu scramble while hot, with the add ons on the ingredient list avocado slices, salsa, nutritional yeast.

Begin your veggie-filled day with this tofu scramble loaded with different colored veggies and behold the health it will bring you.

5.1.8 Avocado and Bean Breakfast Bake

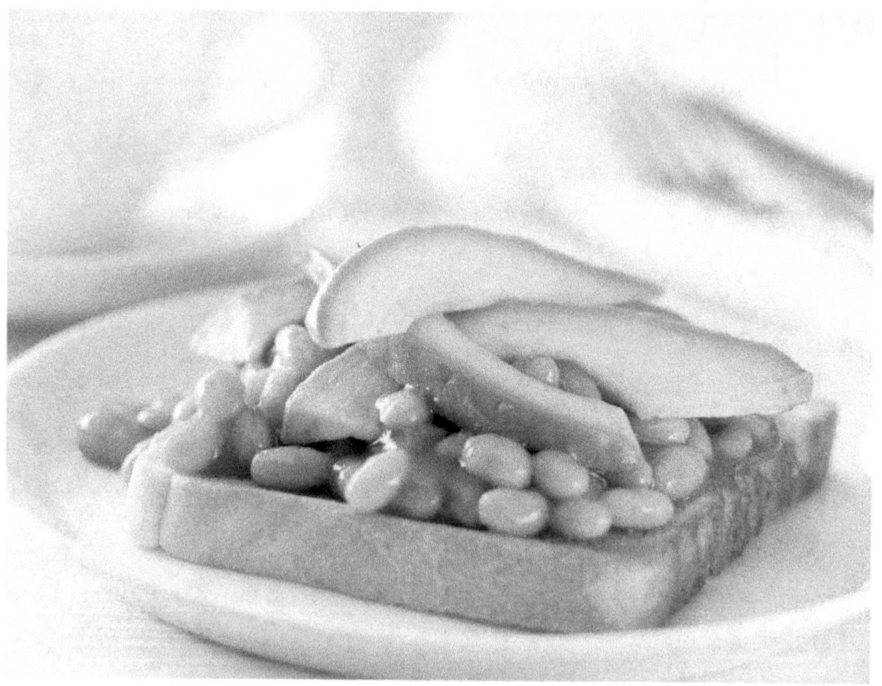

Ingredients:

- 15 oz black beans, drained and rinsed.
- 1 cup cherry tomatoes, halved
- 1 avocado, diced
- 1/2 cup chopped red onion.
- 6 large eggs
- 1/4 cup of milk, either dairy or nondairy.
- 1 teaspoon ground cumin
- 1 teaspoon chili powder

- Salt and pepper to taste
- 1 cup grated cheese (cheddar or Monterey Jack, as preferred).
- Fresh cilantro for garnish (optional)

Instructions:

1. Preheat the oven to 375 °F (190 °C). Coat the baking dish with cooking or olive oil spray.

2. In the meantime in a bowl, add black beans; cherry tomatoes; diced avocado and chopped red onions. Spread this compound onto the greased and lined baking tray evenly.

3. In another bowl mix eggs, milk, ground cumin, chili powder, salt and pepper.

4. Add egg mixture to bean and vegetable mixture, pop in baking dish.

5. Top with shredded cheese.

6. Bake in the preheated oven at 425 degrees F or until the eggs set and top is golden brown for 25-30 minutes.

7. Remove from the oven, let cool slightly and cut.

8. Top with fresh cilantro (optional), and serve hot.

I hope you get tasty when you get Avocado and Bean Breakfast Bake.

5.2 Vegetarian Recipes

5.2.1 Lemon Garlic Shrimp

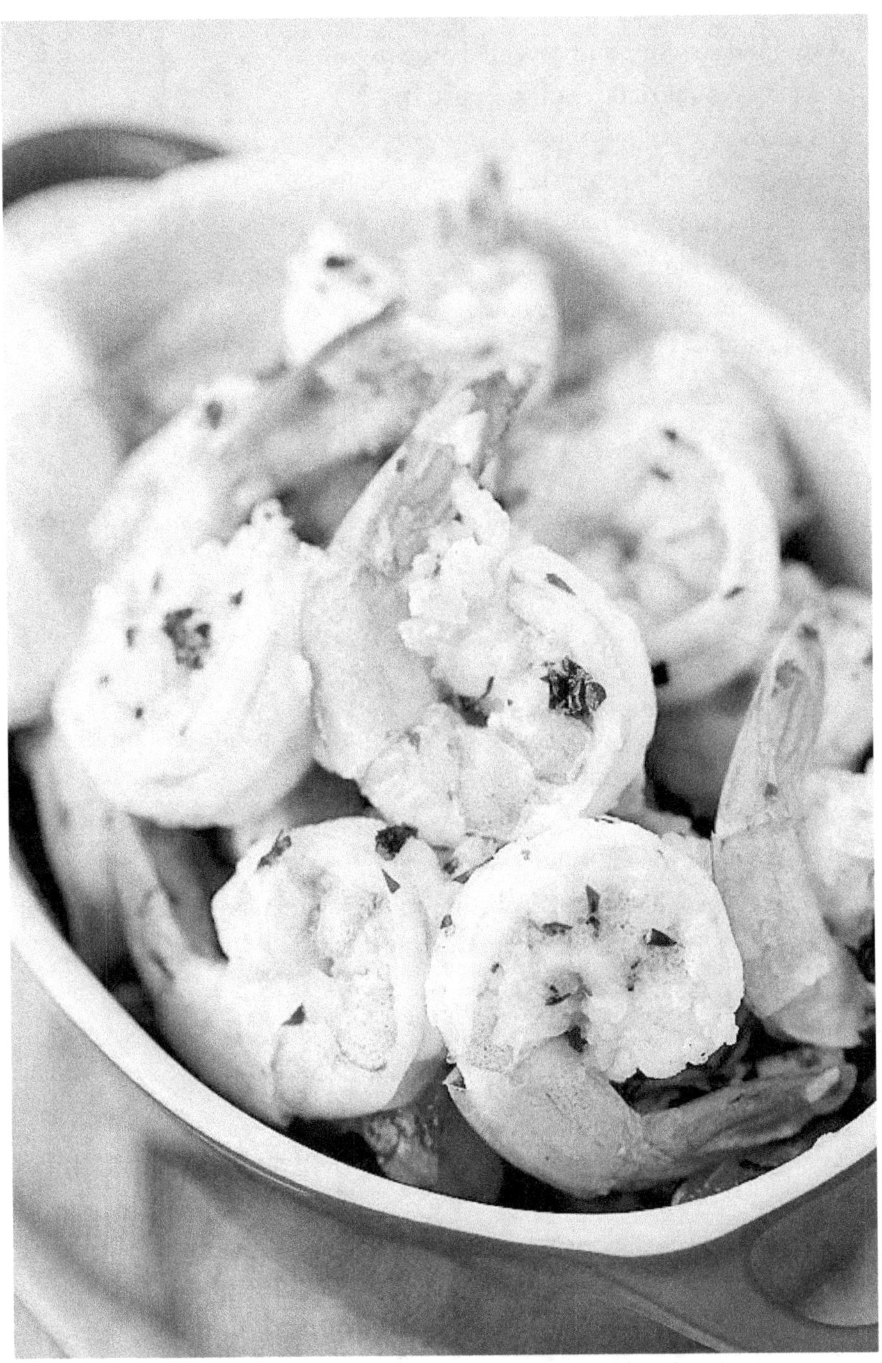

Ingredients:

- 1 pound shell-off and deveined prawns
- 3 tablespoons of olive oil chopped
- 4 garlic cloves
- 1 teaspoon red pepper flakes (or more to taste)
- Lemon juice from one lemon
- zest of 1 lemon
- 2 tablespoons fresh cut parsley
- Salt and black pepper to taste

Instructions:

1. Combine shrimp in bowl along with salt, black pepper, red pepper flakes, sliced garlic and olive oil make sure they are coated thickly.

2. Put a big skillet on high heat.

3. Add the shrimps onto the pan after becoming opaque and pinkish for around two or three minutes either side.

4. After tossing it to mix well with yumminess let it be still for another minute or two so that flavors might intermingle more while the shrimp will be covered by lime juices as you pour over them.

5. A finely chopped fresh parsley would do great when you need to add some freshness into the prawn.

6. Keep tasting until you get what pleases your tongue's buds.

7. In case you may want crispy bread beside it or some rice/pasta underneath feel free to arrange them in that way as an alternative to serve either at your wish.

Enjoy this delicious seafood dish!

5.2.2 Whole Roasted Trout

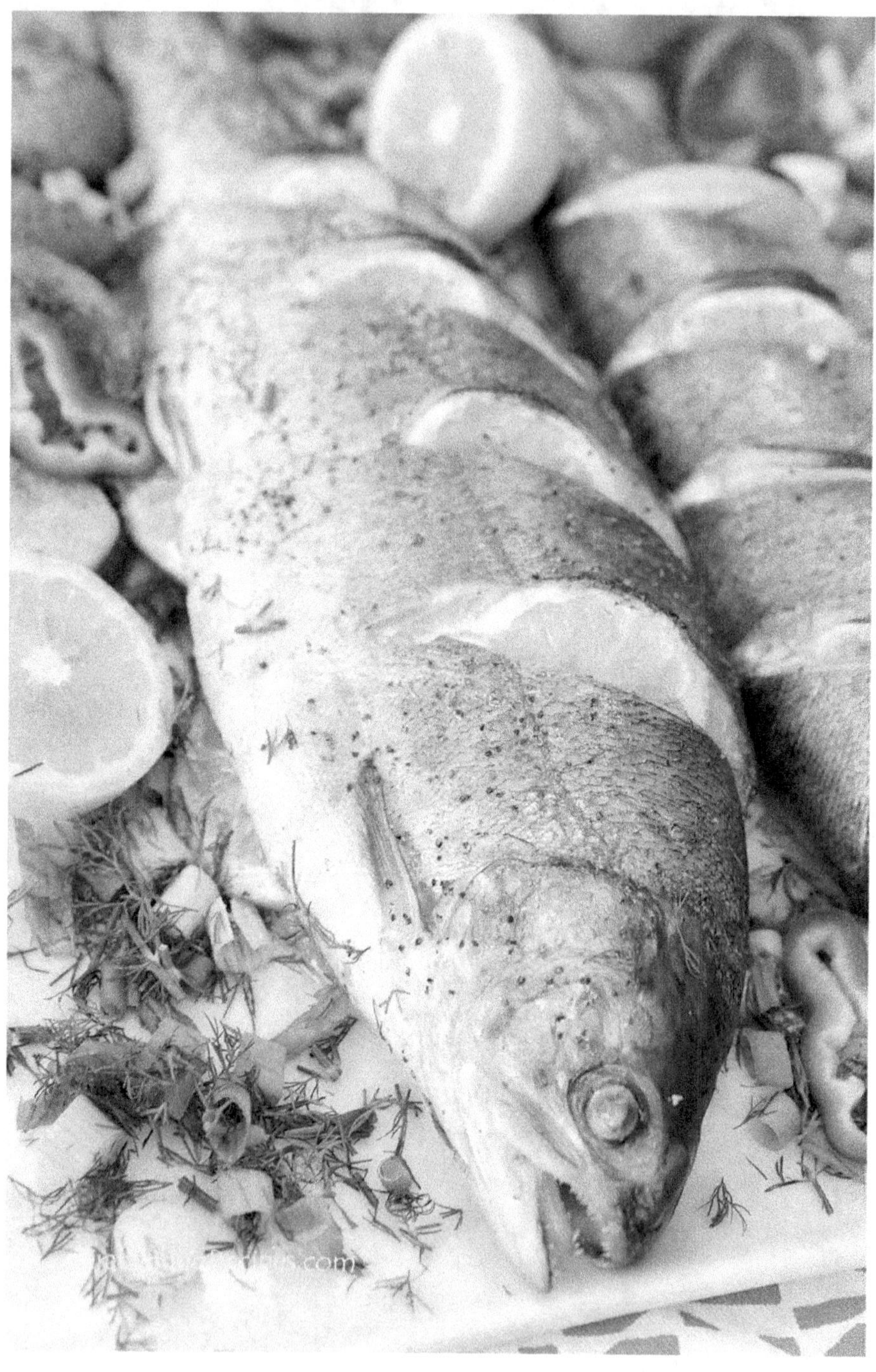

Ingredients:

- 2 whole trout
- 2 oil spoons
- 2 garlic bits
- 1 lemon, thin
- Fresh plant
- Salt, pepper
- Optional: mustard

Instructions:

1. Set the oven temperature to 400°F, or 200°C. Use material paper to line a baking sheet.

2. Use paper towels to wipe dry the fish subsequent to flushing them in cool water.

3. Join olive oil, salt, dark pepper, and cleaved garlic in a little bowl.

4. Apply the olive oil combination to the trout's outside and inside.

5. Embed new spices and lemon cuts into the trout's depression.

6. Optional: For additional flavor, daintily cover the outside of the trout with Dijon mustard.

7. Put the trout onto the baking sheet that has been prepared.

8. Cook the trout for 15 to 20 minutes, or until it chips effectively with a fork, in a preheated stove.

9. For crispier skin, cook for an additional a few minutes, on the off chance

that you'd like.

10. Tenderly put the roasted trout on a plate for show.

11. Add all the more new spices and lemon cuts as embellishment.

Present the whole cooked trout alongside your favored side dishes for a scrumptious and nutritious supper!

5.2.3 Coconut and Kale Fish Curry

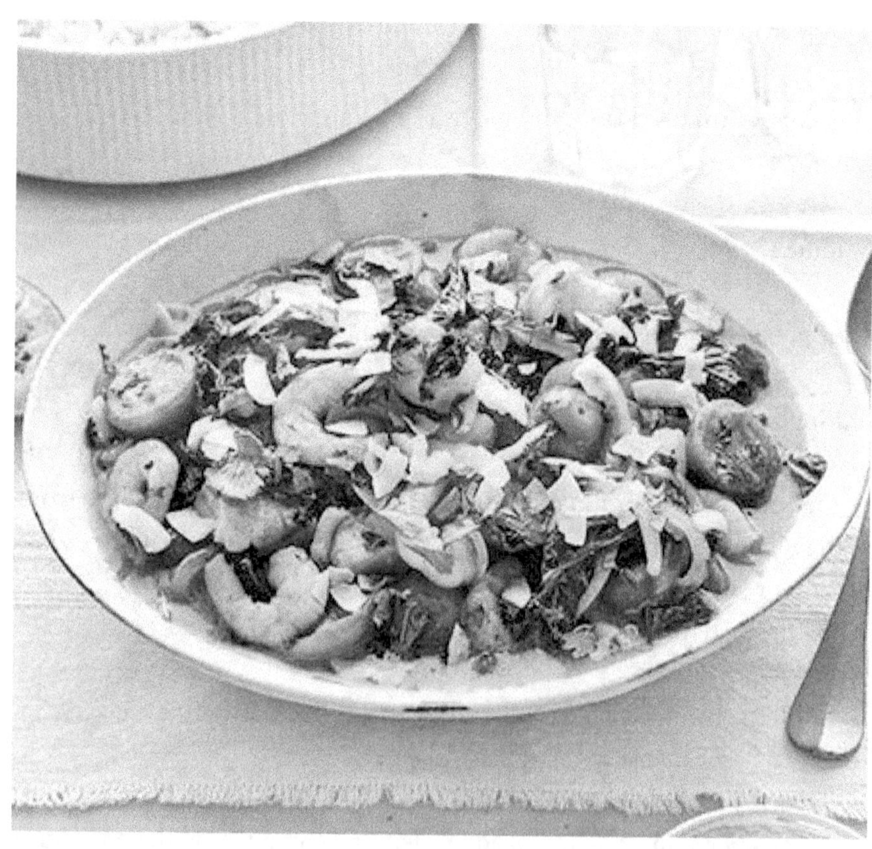

Ingredients:

- 1 pound white fish fillets (such as cod or tilapia), cut into chunks
- 1 can (13.5 oz) coconut milk1 onion, finely chopped
- 3 cloves garlic, minced
- 1 tablespoon ginger, grated
- 1 tablespoon curry powder
- 1 teaspoon ground turmeric
- 1 teaspoon cumin
- 1 teaspoon coriander
- 1/2 teaspoon red pepper flakes (adjust to taste)
- 1 can (14 oz) diced tomatoes, undrained
- 4 cups kale, stems removed and chopped
- Salt and pepper to taste
- Fresh cilantro for garnish
- Cooked rice for serving

Instructions:

1. Heat a little proportion of oil in a significant dish or pot over medium force. The chopped onions should be cooked until they become tender.

2. Grind the ginger and slash the garlic into the onions. Sauté one more moment or so until fragrant.

3. Curry powder, powdered turmeric, cumin, coriander, and red pepper chips should be added. To toast the flavors, cook for a further one to two minutes.

4. Fill the container with cut tomatoes and their juice, close by coconut milk. Mix well to combine.

5. Stew the mix for a short time frame. Add the fish pieces and cook for five

to seven minutes, or until they are almost done.

6. Consolidate the curry with cut greens. Stew until the fish is done and the kale begins to recoil.

7. To taste, add salt and pepper to the curry.

8. Trim with fresh cilantro before serving the coconut and kale fish curry over cooked rice.

5.2.4 Moroccan Seafood Tagine

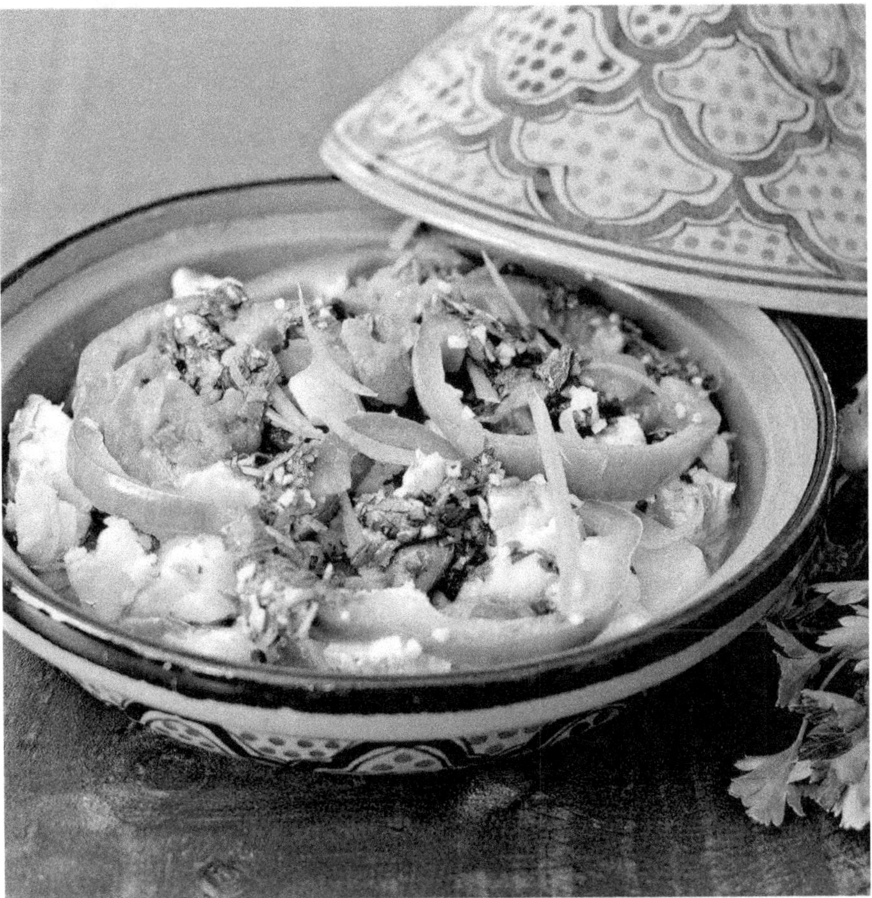

Ingredients:

- 1 pound of arranged seafood, like calamari, mussels, and shrimp.
- 2 teaspoons olive oil - One finely cut onion 3 minced garlic cloves
- 1 teaspoon every one of ground cumin and coriander
- 1 teaspoon of paprika
- A portion of a teaspoon of ground cinnamon
- 1/2 teaspoon cayenne pepper (acclimate to taste) - 1/2 teaspoon powdered turmeric
- One 14-oz container of hacked, undrained tomatoes
- A portion of a cup of vegetable or fish stock

- 1 meagerly cut saved lemon
- A portion of a cup of pitted green olives; New parsley or cilantro for adornment
- To taste, salt and pepper
- Cooked couscous for serving

Instructions:

1. Heat the olive oil in a major container or tajine over medium intensity. Cook the hacked onions until they become delicate.

2. Add the minced garlic and sauté it until fragrant with the onions.

3. Ground paprika, ground cinnamon, ground turmeric, ground cumin, and ground coriander can all be added. Stew for a couple of moments to draw out the smells of the flavors.

4. When the seafood has started to turn misty, add the blended seafood to the flavor combination and stew for a couple of moments.

5. Add the cleaved tomatoes and fish or vegetable stock. Thoroughly mix.

6. Top the tajine with cuts of saved lemon and green olives.

7. When the seafood is cooked through, decrease the intensity to low, cover, and stew for 15 to 20 minutes.

8. To taste, add salt and pepper for preparing.

9. Not long prior to serving, decorate with new parsley or cilantro.

10. Top cooked couscous with Moroccan Seafood Tajine.

Appreciate your tasty and exquisite Moroccan feast!

5.2.5 Chickpea and Vegetable Buddha Bowl

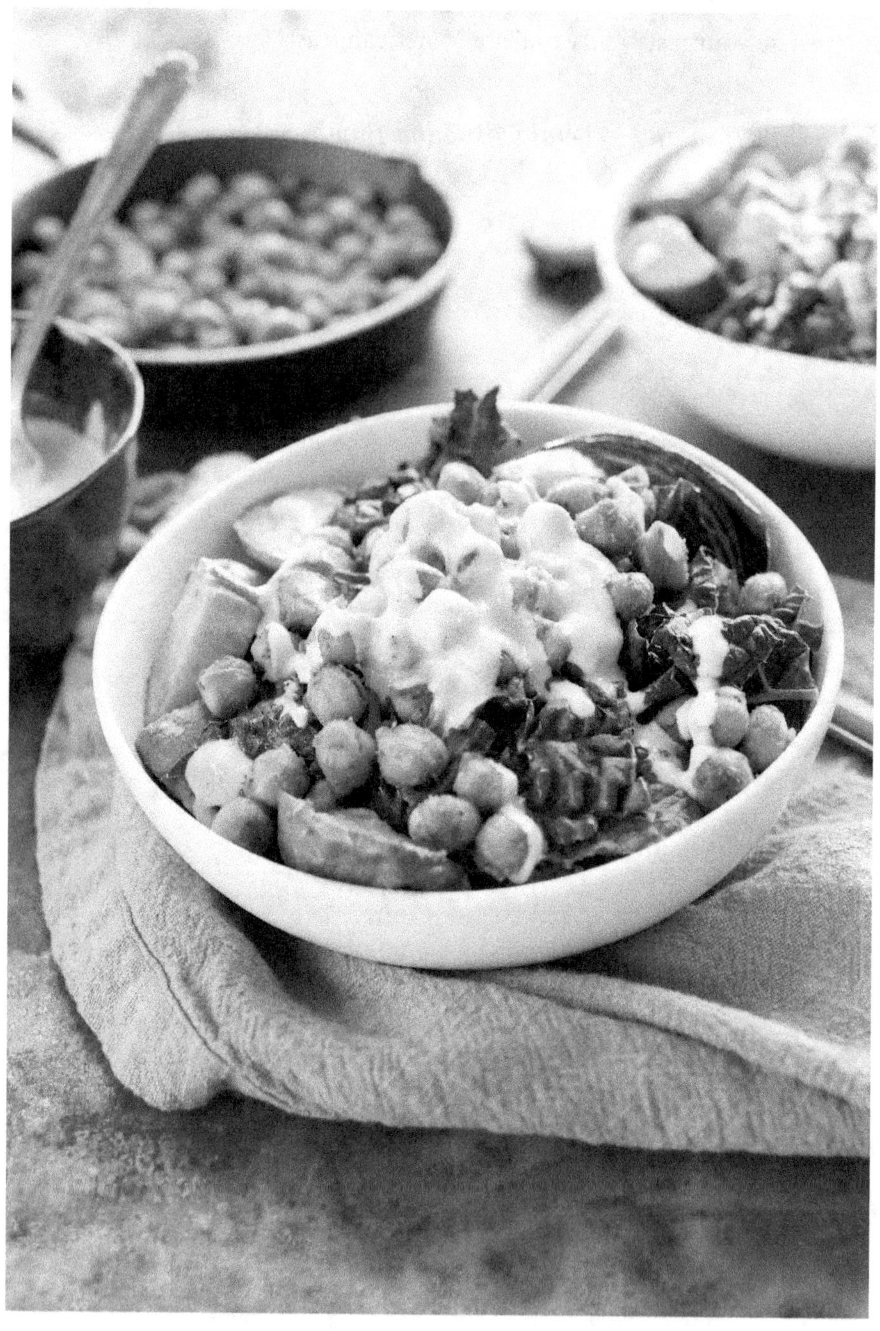

Ingredients

- 1 cup cooked quinoa or brown rice
- 1 cup chickpeas (canned, drained, and rinsed)
- 1 cup mixed vegetables (e.g., broccoli, bell peppers, cherry tomatoes)
- 1 tablespoon olive oil
- 1 teaspoon smoked paprika
- 1/2 teaspoon cumin
- Salt and pepper to taste
- Avocado slices for topping
- Greek yogurt or tahini for drizzling
- Fresh herbs (cilantro or parsley) for garnish

Instructions:

1. Set the oven's temperature to 200°C, or 400°F.

2. Add the chickpeas, olive oil, smoked paprika, salt, and pepper to the vegetables that have been pureed.

3. Put the chickpeas and vegetables on a baking sheet and dish for 20 to 25 minutes, or until the veggies are delicate.

4. While the rice or quinoa is cooking, orchestrate it as indicated by the holder's bearings.

5. To collect your Buddha bowl, place a piece of cooked quinoa or natural hued rice in a dish.

6. Orchestrate the veggies and broiled chickpeas on top.

7. Add avocado cuts and tahini or Greek yogurt up and over.

8. Add a few new spices as an enhancement.

5.2.6 Sweet Potato and Black Bean Stuffed Peppers

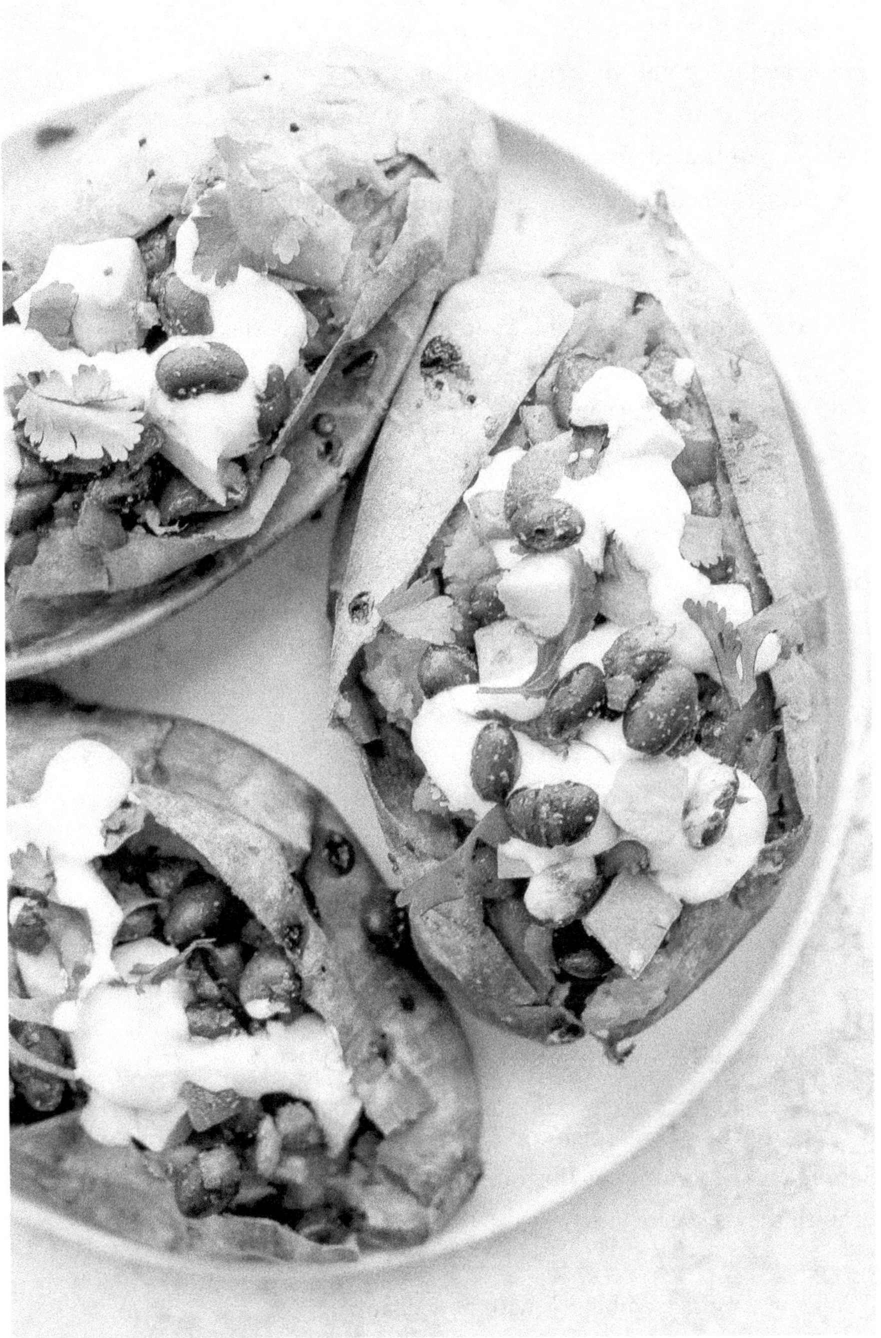

Ingredients:

- 1 can (15 oz) of washed and depleted dark beans
- 2 medium potatoes, stripped and diced
- 4 enormous ringer peppers, cut down the middle and cultivated
- 1 cup of tinned, frozen, or new corn parts
- 1 cup slashed tomatoes, either canned or fresh
- 1 teaspoon chili powder
- 1/2 smoked paprika
- 1 cup of destroyed cheddar (either cheddar or a Mexican mix)
- Salt and pepper to taste
- Fresh cilantro for garnish
- Salsa or Greek yogurt to serve

Instructions:

1. Turn the oven on to 375°F, or 190°C.

2. Move the halved pepper parts to a baking plate.

3. Consolidate the diced potatoes, dark beans, corn, diced tomatoes, cumin, smoked paprika, stew powder, and salt and pepper in a major bowl.

4. Stuff the potatoes and dark bean blend into every portion of a chime pepper.

5. Sprinkle shredded cheese over the stuffed peppers

6. Prepare the baking dish for 25 to 30 minutes while covered with foil. Subsequent to eliminating the foil, bakel the peppers for a further 10 minutes, or until they are delicate.

7. Whenever liked, embellish with new cilantro.

8. Spread salsa or Greek yogurt on top of the peppers that have been served.

5.2.7 Seafood Delight Paella

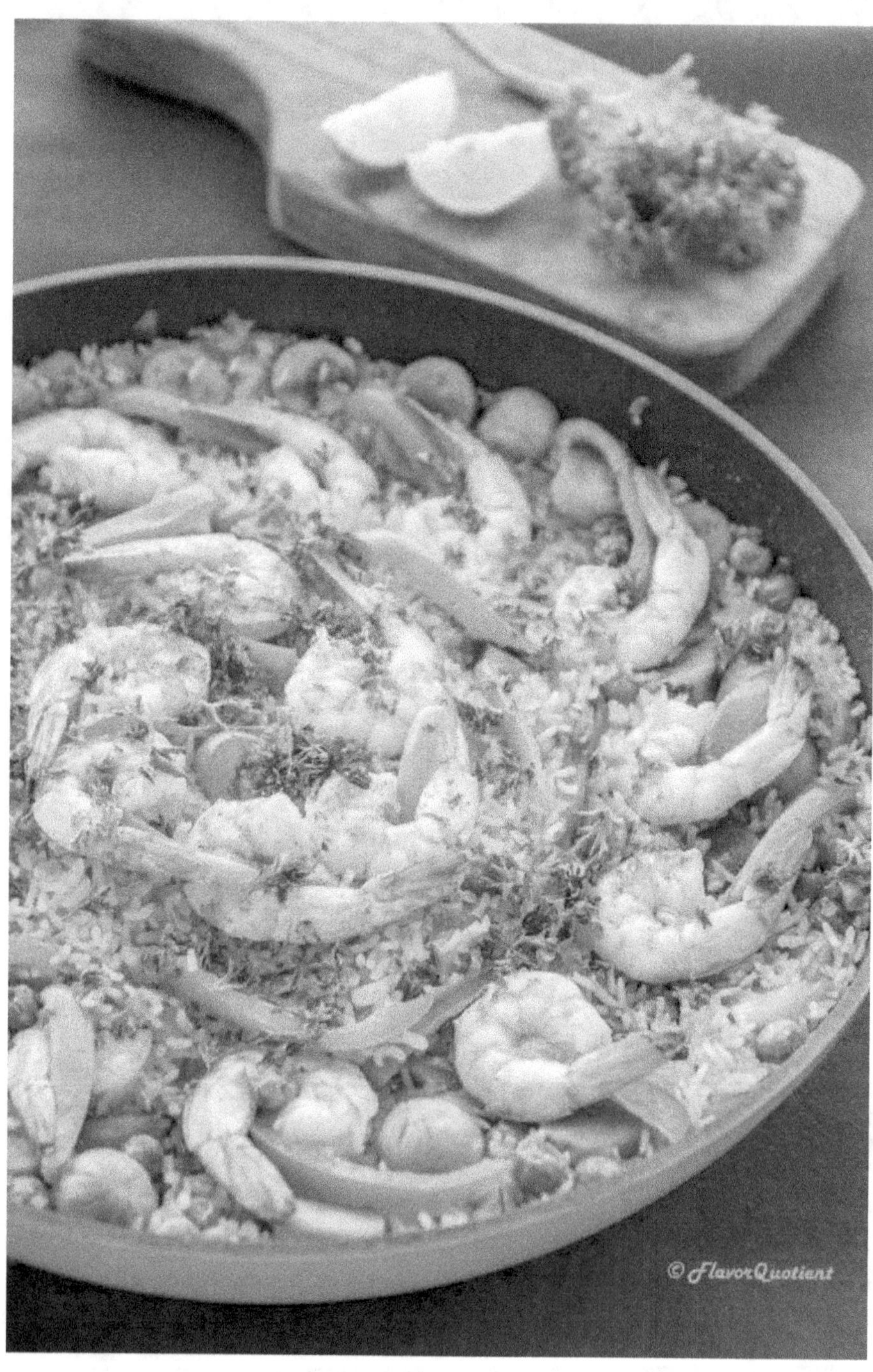

Ingredients:

- 1 and 1/2 cups Arborio or short-grain rice.
- About 1 lb of mixed seafood ((shrimp/mussels/clams/squid) already cleaned and ready-to-eat).
- 1/2 cup cooked, shelled crab.
- 1 onion, finely chopped
- 3 cloves garlic, minced
- 1 red bell pepper, sliced
- 1 tomato, diced
- 1/2 cup frozen peas
- 4 vegan fish/ vegetable stock.
- 1/2 cup white wine
- Watered saffron, 1 tsp saffron threads
- 1 teaspoon smoked paprika
- Salt and pepper to taste
- 1/4 cup fresh parsley, chopped
- Lemon wedges for serving

Instructions:

1. In a paella pan or large skillet fry vegetable oil on medium heat. Incorporate diced onions and simmer.

2. Add garlic and sauteed with onions till fragrant.

3. Add red pepper and as an option put diced tomato. Not more than two minutes should be used before even some of the vegetables start to get soft.

4. In the pan add the Arborio rice and stir to make sure every grain soaks in vegetable mixture.

5. Mix the white wine after that let simmering the mixture for a few minutes, until most of the wine evaporates.

6. In a skillet, put in saffron threads and the water used to infuse it, smoked paprika, salt and pepper Stir to combine.

7. Add the broth and simmer the content. Reduce heat to medium-low.

8. Distribute the sea mix, crab meat and frozen peas evenly across the rice. Do not stray away from this stage for the last act of bamboo zombies is not to let the crust formative the bottom.

9. Let cook under moderately high heat for 20 to 25 minutes and when the rice is tender and the water is absorbed, turn the heat off. When need be, spill in some other spoons of broth.

10. Remove from the heat, cover with a clean kitchen towel; leave for 5 minutes.

11. Garnish with freshly chopped parsley and accompany with lemon wedges.

5.3 Healthy Snack Recipes for IF

5.3.1 Baked Sweet Potato Chips

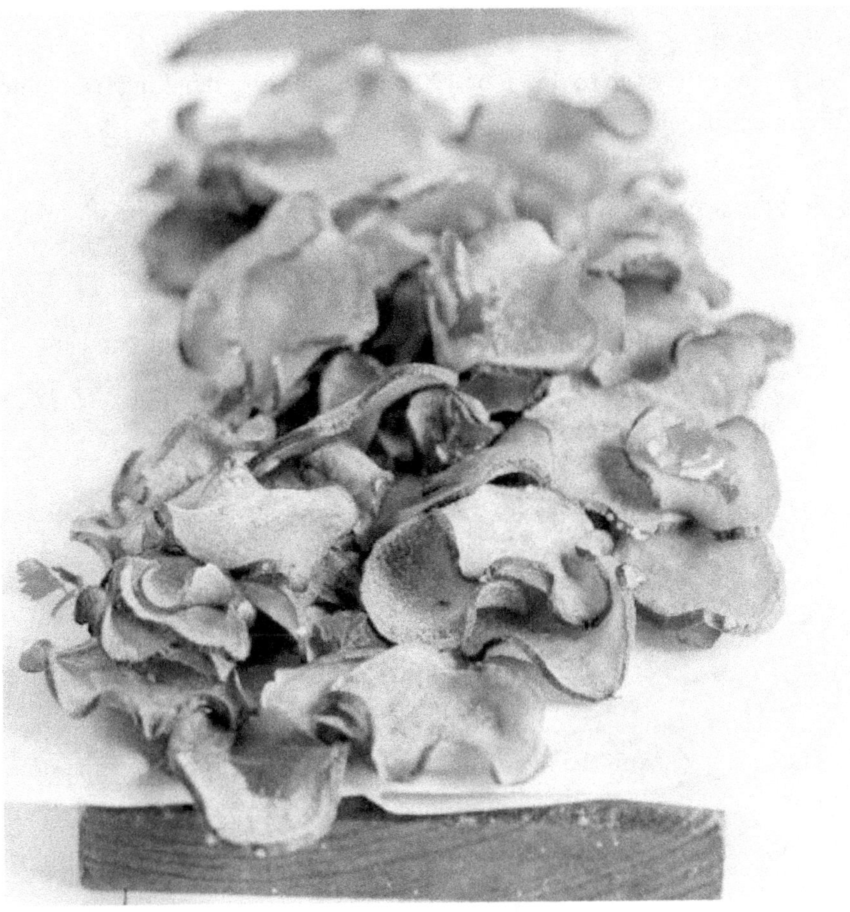

Ingredients:

- 2 medium – sized sweet potatoes washed and peeled.
- 2 tablespoons olive oil
- 1 teaspoon paprika
- 1/2 teaspoon garlic powder
- 1/2 TV leaf of salt (Add according to the smell).
- 1/4 teaspoon black pepper
- Optional: for some heat, add a pinch of cayenne pepper.

Instructions:

1. Preheat the oven to 375°F or 190°C. On the second baking trays, line parchment paper.

2. Peel the sweet potatoes, cut them slice using either a mandoline slicer or a sharp knife to get round, thin slices.

3. Add the sweet potato slices to a large bowl, mix them with olive oil and all the seasonings – paprika, garlic powder, salt, pepper as well as black pepper. Make sure they are coated in your mix thoroughly.

4. Lay the sweet potato slices that have been spiced in the prepared baking pans, one layer, not touching and not overlapping each other.

5. Bake chips for 15-20 minutes on the preheated oven flip halfway to get perfect golden brown and crunchy. Just keep an eye if they burn.

6. Then remove from the oven and let the baked sweet potato chips stick a little while to cool on the baking sheets. Once they cool, they will keep crisping.

7. Then one can transfer the chips to a serving bowl; chips are a healthy snack.

5.3.2 Crispy Kale Chips

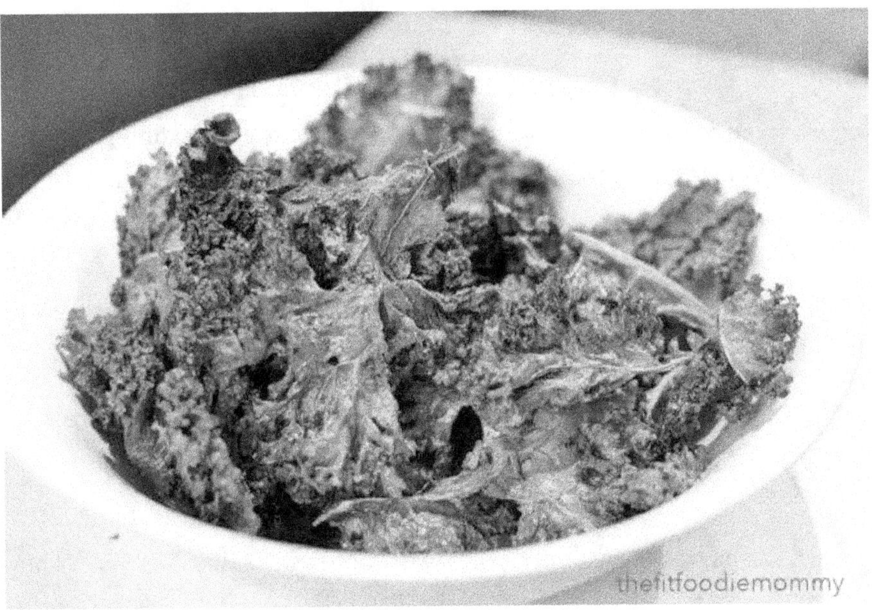

Ingredients:

- 1 bunch (typically 6-8 cups) of fresh kale.
- 1 tablespoon of olive oil and garlic powder.
- 1/2 teaspoon of powdered onion.
- ½ smoked paprika
- Season to taste, with salt, and pepper.

Instructions:

1. Warm your oven to 150° C or 300° F . Arrange the paper on the 2 nd baking tray.

2. Rinse and wash the kale leaves rather well then dry them gently using clean kitchen towels or paper towels.

3. First tear the rough stems off the leaves of kale and chop it into manageable

pieces.

4. To a large bowl add olive oil, salt, pepper, smoky paprika, onion powder and garlic powder and toss in kale pieces. Uniformly cover all leaves.

5. In order to prevent the disorderly overlapping of the kale pieces, the kale leaves should be symmetrical laid out into a single layer over the roasting dishes/trays.

6. For 15 to 20 minutes, bake until the kale is brittle with just a tinge of color. Observe so that they do not burn.

7. Take the baking sheets out of the oven and let the kale chips cool. They will get crispy as they cool.

8. What is more, transfer kale chips to a serving dish and it becomes the perfect healthy and yummy snack.

This is a kale chips crispy and healthy vacation session. Feel free to adjust the seasonings to your taste. Have fun!

5.3.3 Spiced Nuts

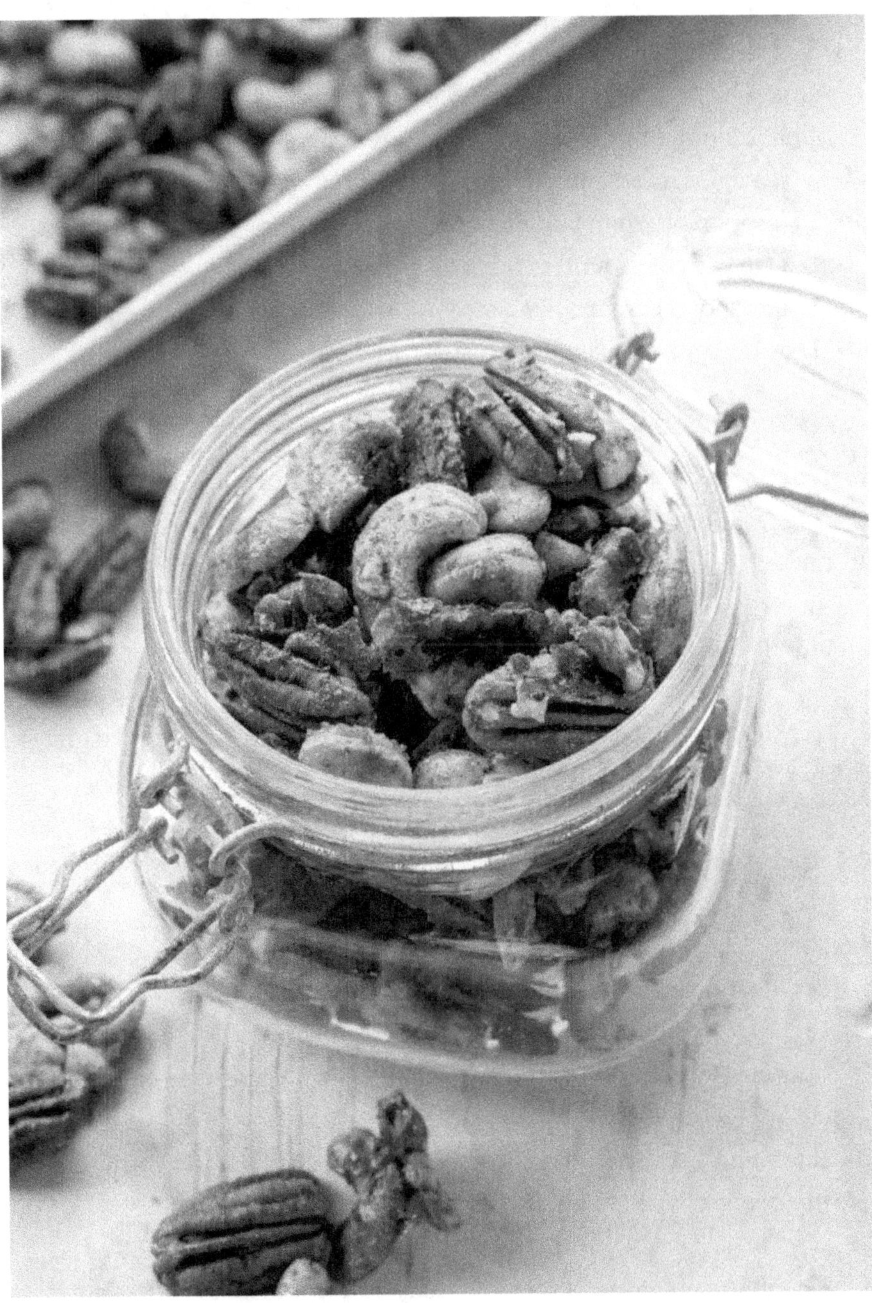

Ingredients:

- 2 cups of combined nuts which include cashews, pecans, walnuts, and almonds
- 1 tablespoon of melted butter over olive oil
- 2 teaspoons honey/maple syrup.
- 1 teaspoon of ground cinnamon
- 1/2 tsp each of ground cumin and smoked paprika
- 1/4 teaspoon cayenne pepper
- 1/2 tablespoon of salt (or to taste).

Instructions:

1. Increase to 325°F, or 900°C. Inside the tray, cut the parchment paper around.

2. Add the honey together with the melted butter/olive oil into a big bowl.

3. Transfer the mixed nuts to the bowl, shake well to coat the nuts in the entire mixture.

4. Mixed ground cumin, ground cinnamon, smoked paprika, cayenne pepper, and salt.

5. Toss the nuts in one last time after the salt is mixed in to evenly coat.

6. Put some spiced nuts on an even surface onto the prepared baking sheet.

7. Bake the nuts for 15 to 20 minutes in the oven at 175 degrees or until they become fragrant and are all toasted in a uniform manner.

8. Take out the spiced nuts from the oven and allow them to cool completely on the baking sheet. Since they cool, they will be crispy.

9. Cool the nuts after they are roasted; then refrigerate them in a sealed

container.

Enjoy the taste of your home-made spiced nuts with the right balance of sweetness, crunch, and spice as a sumptuous filler.

5.3.4 home-made Granola Bars

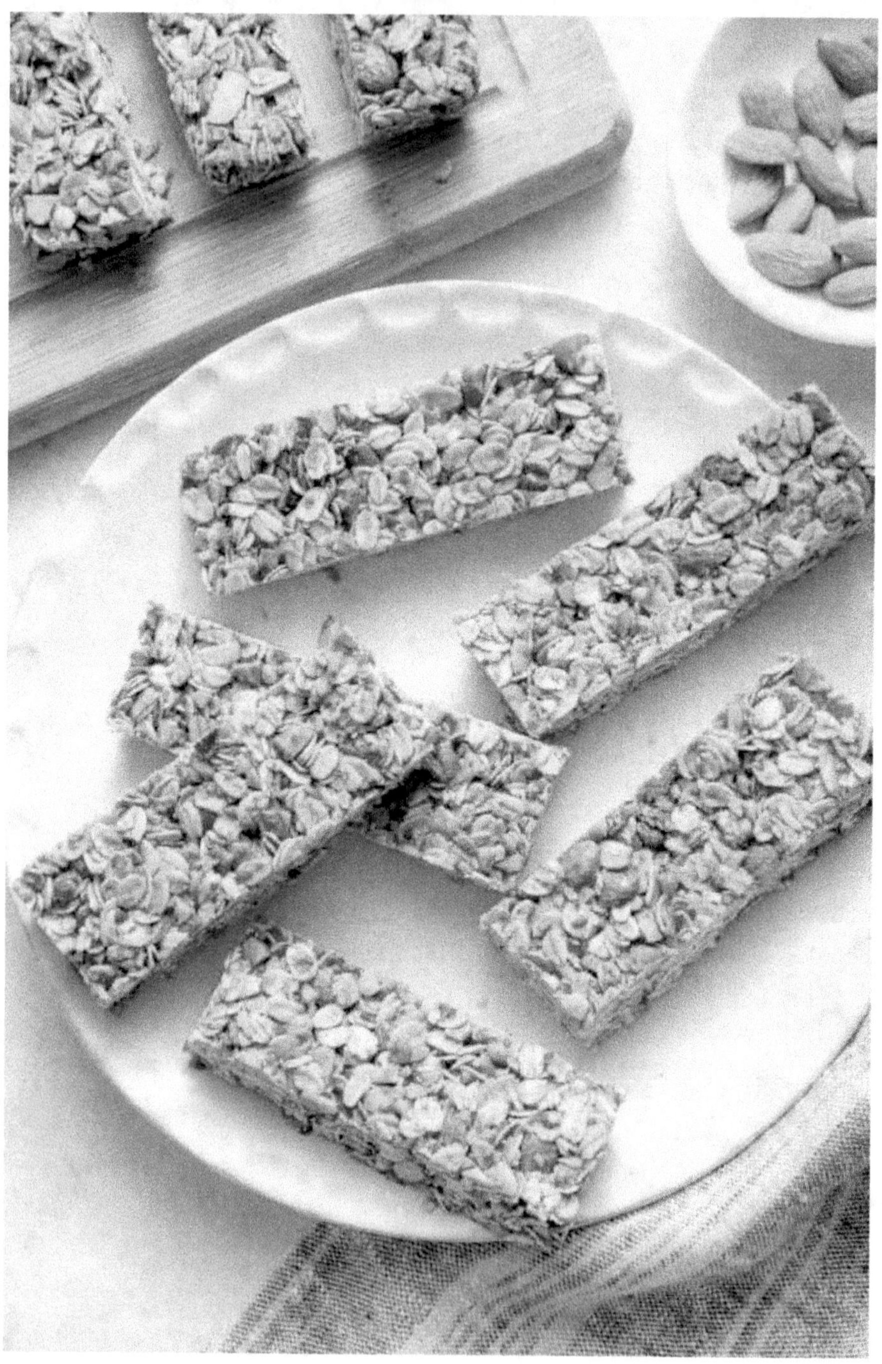

Ingredients:

- 2 cups of old-fashioned oats.
- Chopped one cup nuts (almonds, walnuts or your choice)
- 1/2 cup of honey or maple syrup.
- Nut butter, unsweetened, in an amount sufficient for 1/4 cup
- 1/4 cup melted coconut oil.
- 1 ml vanilla essence
- Chop any 1/2 cup of dried fruit (raisins, cranberries, apricots, ect.)
- 1/4 tablespoon salt (optional).

Instructions:

1. Heat your oven to 350°F (175°C) preheat.Allow parchment paper to hang, some overhang on the sides, to facilitate easy removal of the mixture with the utensil.

2. Top oats and chopped nuts off in a large mixing bowl.

3. In a small saucepan over low heat, bring to a simmer the honey or maple syrup, nut butter, and melted coconut oil.

4. Take the saucepan aside from the stove top and add the vanilla extract to it and mix in; let it cool for a moment.

5. Combine the contents of the mixing bowl – the wet mixture of oats and nuts.Stir until everything is caked.

6. Add the chopped dried fruit and, if you like, some salt for an undertone of savouriness.

7. Fold the mixture of the contents into the previously arranged baking dish. Ease the mixture with a spatula until you flatten it with firmness ensuring even spreading.

8. Do not forget to bake for about 20-25 minutes in a preheated oven until the sides turn golden brown.

9. Once waiting for the granola bars to cool, let it cool thoroughly in the baking dish.

10. Once cooled, pull the parchment paper overhang to lift the bars from the pan.Lemons are to be placed on its cutting board and then cut into bars and squares.

11. Place the granola bars that you have made yourself in an airtight container so they can keep it at room temperature.

Make sure you eat the home-made granola bars that are so good and will provide you with the necessary nutrients.Keep in mind to adjust them according to your taste by adding your favorite nuts, seeds, or dried fruits.

5.3.5 Avocado and Tomato Salsa Rice Cakes

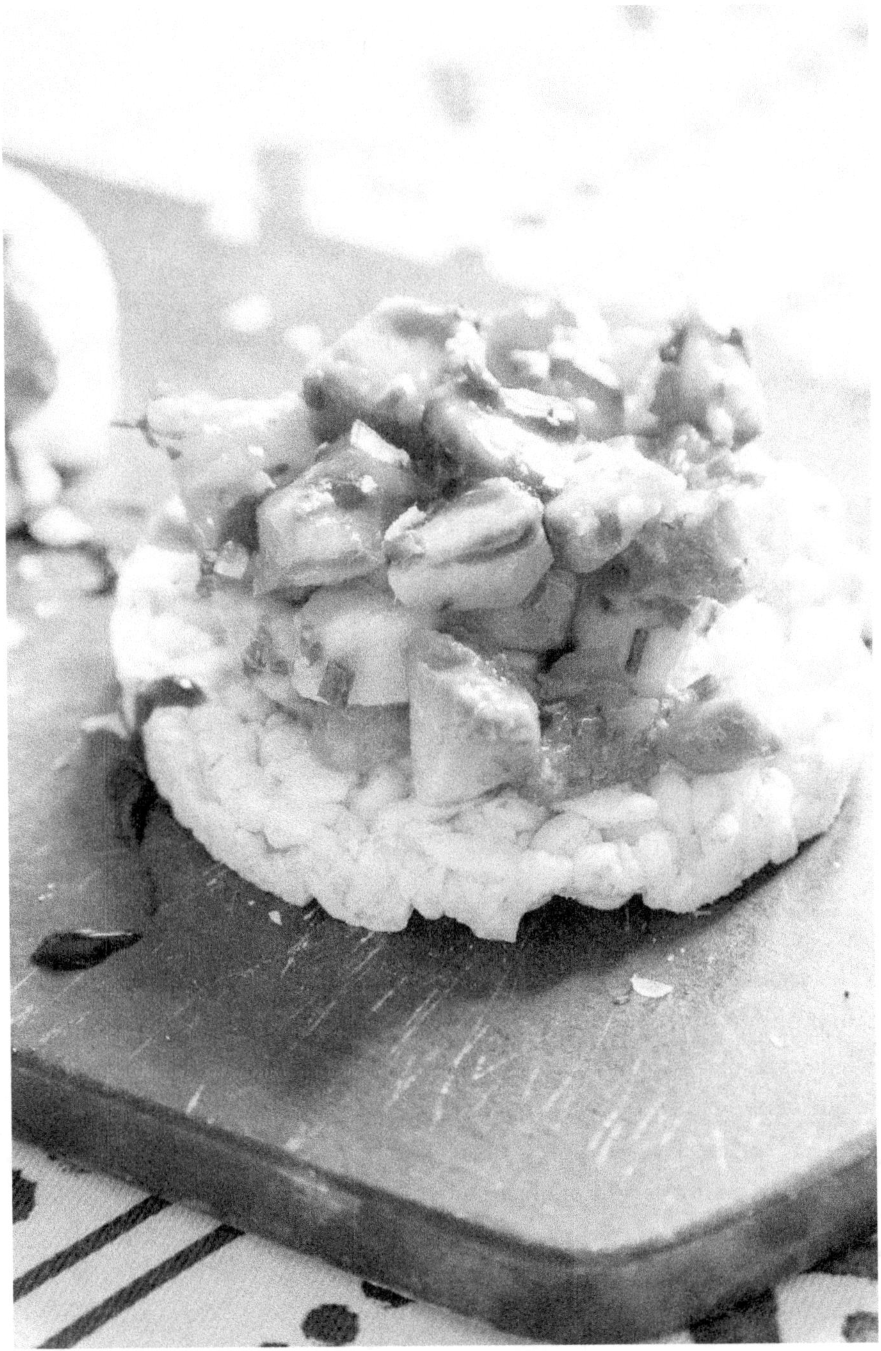

Ingredients:

- 2 rice cakes (with whole grains or with brown rice).
- 1 ready to use avocado mashed.
- One small tomato, diced
- 1/4 red onion - finely chopped.
- 1 tablespoon of fresh cilantro, chopped
- The juice of a half lime
- Season with salt and pepper to your liking
- Optional: As far as I am concerned, a pinch of red pepper flakes is added to make the taste a bit spicy.

Ingredients:

1. The avocado, tomato, red onion, cilantro, lime juice, salt and pepper should be mixed together in a bowl. This is a moderately spicy recipe. If you can stand a little bit of spicy heat to complement the spices, go ahead and sprinkle some chili flakes.

2. In the meantime, toast the rice cakes till they become crisp.

3. The mixture of the mashed avocado and tomato salsa should be spread over the rice cakes coating them entirely.

4. It can also be garnished with additional cilantro or a dash of lime juice, that is optional.

5. Dig in and enjoy this vitamin-rich snack treat.

In between your intermittent fasting period, this Avocado and Tomato Salsa Rice Cakes pellet allows you to satisfy your hunger by incorporating healthy fats, fiber, and vitamins.

5.3.6 Spirulina Popcorn Recipe

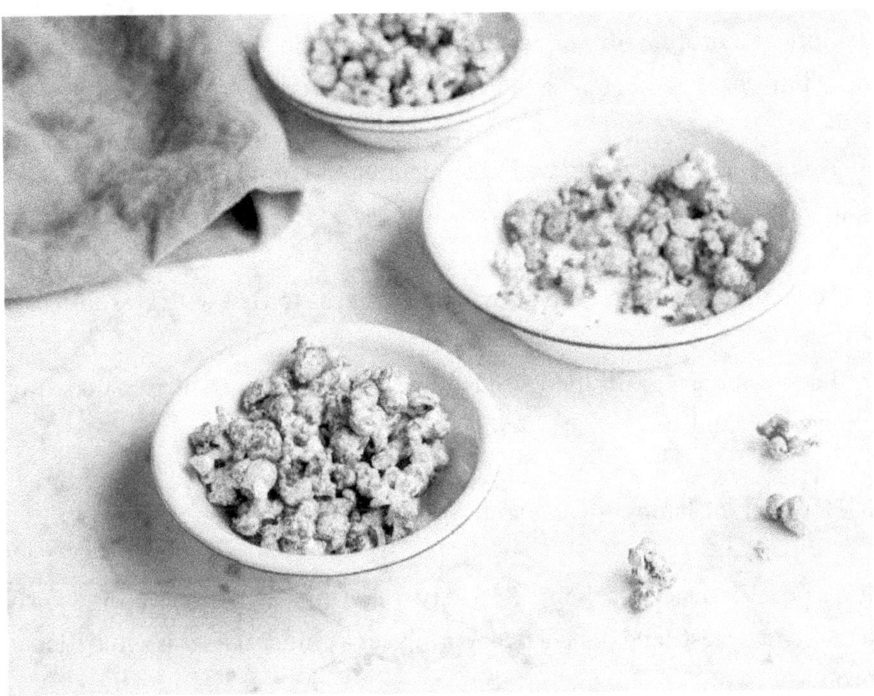

Ingredients:

- 1/2 cup of popcorn kernels
- 2 tbsp coconut oil
- 1-2 teaspoons spirulina powder
- The nutritional yeast, optional to add flavor, is 1 tablespoon

Instructions:

1. Air pop, stovetop pop, or microwave pop your popcorn kernels.In a large bowl, set aside.

2. Add the coconut oil to a small saucepan, and melt over low heat.

3. As melted add the spirulina powder and mix until well incorporated.Also, if you are using nutritional yeast, add it to the mixture.

4. Spread spirulina mixture over the popped popcorn to ensure an even distribution.

5. Toss the popcorn gently with the spirulina mixture.Fold through using a spatula or if cooled slightly, use your hands.

6. Add a pinch of salt on top of the popcorn, toss to coat with seasoning.

7. Each popcorn grain then needs to be cooled and its spirulina coating allowed to solidify.

8. However, be happy and eat your Spirulina Popcorn!

It is a peculiar snack that 's made up of two elements that are spirulina, which has an earthy taste and popcorn that produces a crunch, and it is a nutritional product.

5.3.7 Quinoa Salad Cups

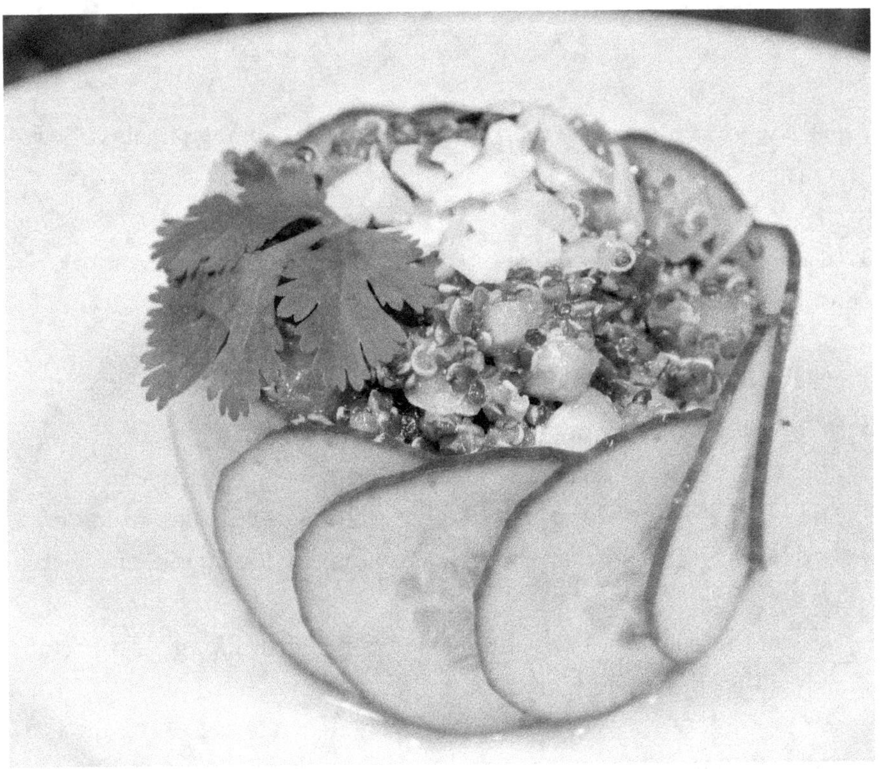

Ingredients:

- 1 cup cooked quinoa, cooled
- Cherry tomatoes, halved
- Cucumber, diced
- Red onion, finely chopped
- Kalamata olives, sliced
- Feta cheese, crumbled
- Fresh basil or mint, choppedOlive oil
- Lemon juice
- Salt and pepper to taste

Instructions:

1. Cook 1/2 cup quinoa, as per the package instructions. Let it cool down

totally.

2. Salad ingredients – halve cherry tomatoes, dice cucumber, finely chop red onion, and slice Kalamata olives.

3. In a big bowl, mix the cold quinoa with cherry tomatoes, cucumber, red onion, Kalamata olives, and feta cheese.

4. Chop basil or mint and add it to the salad to create a flavor punch. Both herb for those who may prefer, and both can be used combined.

5. The salad should be topped with olive oil for a healthy fat. To achieve a zesty dressing, squeeze fresh lemon juice. Combine the ingredients well.

6. Season the salad with salt and pepper as per your liking. If the feta is already salted, be careful with the salt.

7. Divide the quinoa salad into small cups or bowls. This not only simplifies portion control but also provides an attractive appearance.

8. If desired, garnish the cups with some more fresh herbs or a pinch of feta cheese.

These Quinoa Salad Cups are a great snack, light and healthy, during your intermittent fasting window.

It is up to you to modify the recipe by adding other vegetables, protein sources (chickpeas or grilled chicken, for instance), or by changing the herbs and dressing to your liking.

5.4 Smoothies and Beverages Recipe

5.4.1 Cinnamon and Ginger Detox Tea

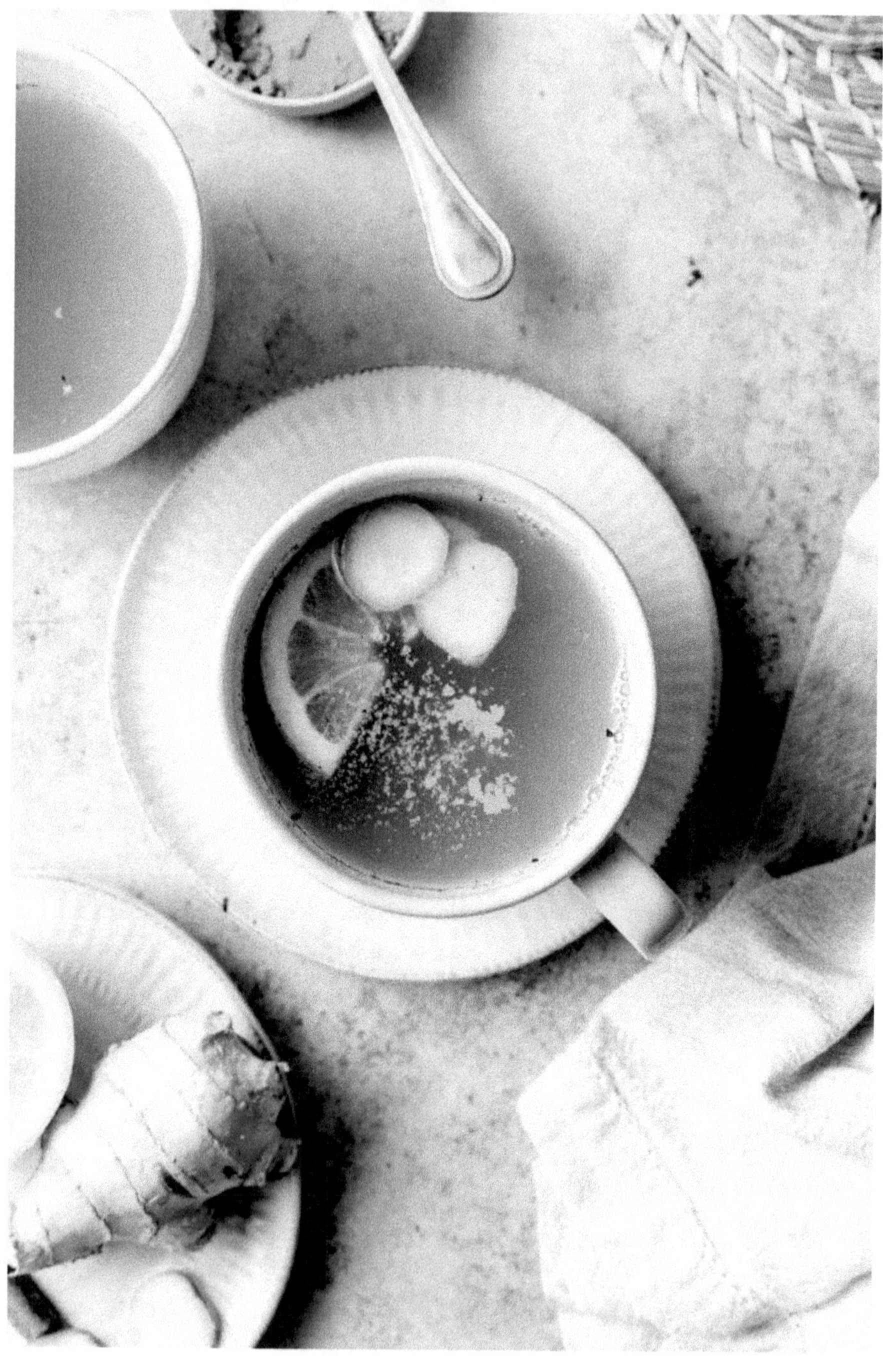

Ingredients:

- 1 inch of freshly peeled and sliced ginger
- 1 tablespoon raw honey (optional) - One cinnamon stick or one teaspoon powdered cinnamon
- ½ a lemon's juice
- 4 cups of water

Instructions:

1. Prepare Ginger: Cut and peel a fresh ginger root, about 1 inch in length. You can add extra slices if you'd like the ginger taste to be stronger.

2. Boil Water: Fill a saucepan with 4 cups of water and bring it to a boil.

3. Add Ginger and Cinnamon: Add the ground cinnamon or a cinnamon stick, along with the slices of ginger, to the saucepan after the water has boiled.

4. Simmer: Lower the heat to a simmer and allow the mixture to cook for ten to fifteen minutes. As a result, the tastes might seep into the water.

5. Strain: After the tea has simmered, strain it to get rid of the chunks of ginger and cinnamon. A tea infuser or a fine-mesh strainer can be used.

6. Sweeten (Optional): You may sweeten the tea with a spoonful of raw honey if you'd like. Until the honey dissolves, stir.

7. Incorporate Lemon Juice: Press the contents of a half-lemon into the tea. Mix thoroughly.

8. Serve: Transfer the cleansing tea into mugs and savor it hot.

The anti-inflammatory and antioxidant qualities of ginger and cinnamon make this Cinnamon and Ginger Detox Tea tasty in addition to perhaps offering health advantages. Savor it as a calming and purifying drink!

5.4.2 Home-made Kombucha

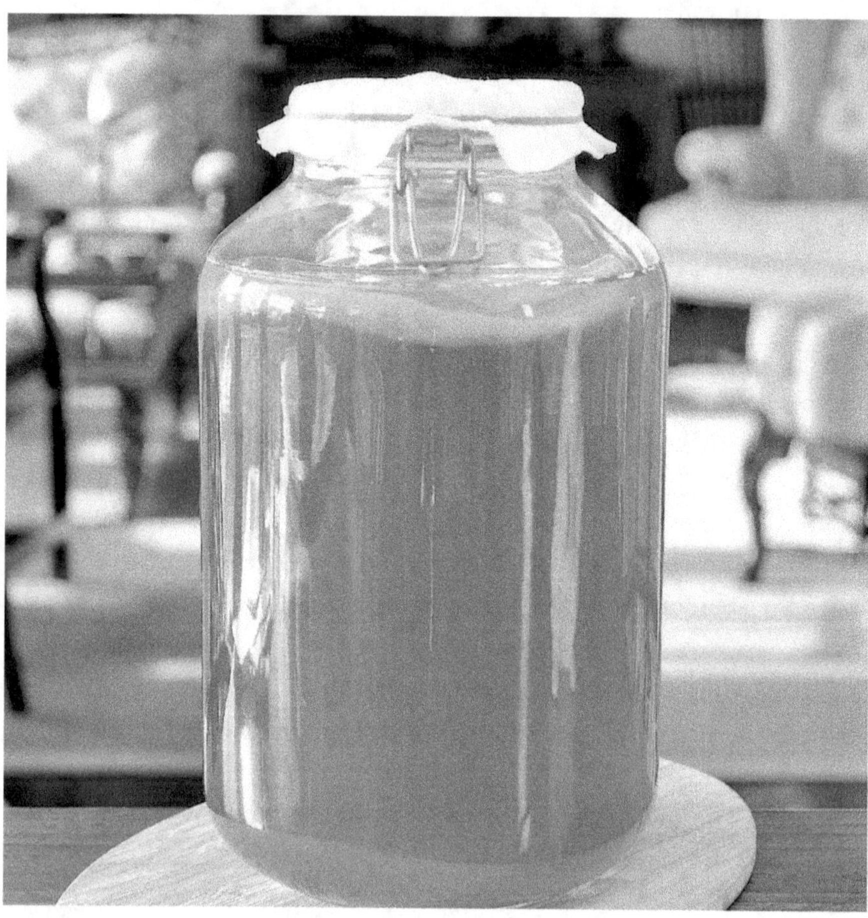

Sweetened tea fermentation using a SCOBY (Symbiotic Culture of Bacteria and Yeast) followed by kombucha flavoring are two fundamental stages of home kombucha production. Here is a simple recipe to get you going:

Ingredients

For the Tea Base:

- 1 gallon or four liters of water
- 4-6 tea bags (green, black, or both).
- The half a cup of sugar shredded.

For the Fermentation Process:

- Could be SCOBY, bought or recovered from a previous batch.
- 1-2 cups of initiation tea (liquid from the previous batch or raw and unflavored kombucha available through commercials).

Instructions:

1. Prepare the Tea Base:

- Put the sugar and tea bags in a vast amount of boiled water.
- The tea is required to steep for anywhere between ten and fifteen minutes after stirring to ensure the sugar dissolves.
- While it is still hot, let the tea cool until it attains room temperature.

2. Mix the starter tea, SCOBY, and tea base together:

- The latter is an effective mechanism to protect companies from dubious parties.
- Transfer the chilled out tea into a large clean glass recipient.
- Secondly,mate is store bought kombucha or starter tea from a previous batch.
- Add the SCOBY carefully above the liquid.

3. Cover and Ferment:

- Covering the jar with fresh cloth or coffee filter, the jar then is tightened with a rubber band.
- Through the same considerations, if you like the color, leave the jar in warm dark place between 70°F and 75°F (21° –24°C) fermenting between 7 and 30 days.

4. Check Fermentation:

- Taste the kombucha after two or three days. Once acidity and sweetness measures have been reached, it is ready to move to the next phase.

5: Strain Out SCOBY:

- The SCOBY will have to be gently taken out of the jar and placed in a sanitized container.

6. At this point you can add flavor to your kombucha. It may well be applied to fruits, spices, or even plants.

Some of the kombucha should remain at the top when you pour it into the smaller bottles.

7. Second Fermentation:

- Once the bottles are sealed, let the ones ferment for 3 to 7 days at room temperature. Secondly, this facilitates the carbonation of the kombucha.

8. Refrigerate and Enjoy:

- Place the bottles in a glass refrigerator to stop fermentation, once the desired level of carbonation is attained.
- With your kombucha being home-made , enjoy the cold kombucha as early as you can!

Note: To avoid contracting infections, always ensure you are using clean jars and utensils. It furthermore includes avoidance of metal utensils and containers which can interact with the kombucha. More importantly, be careful throughout the process as well as hygiene.

5.4.3 Green Pineapple Coconut Smoothie

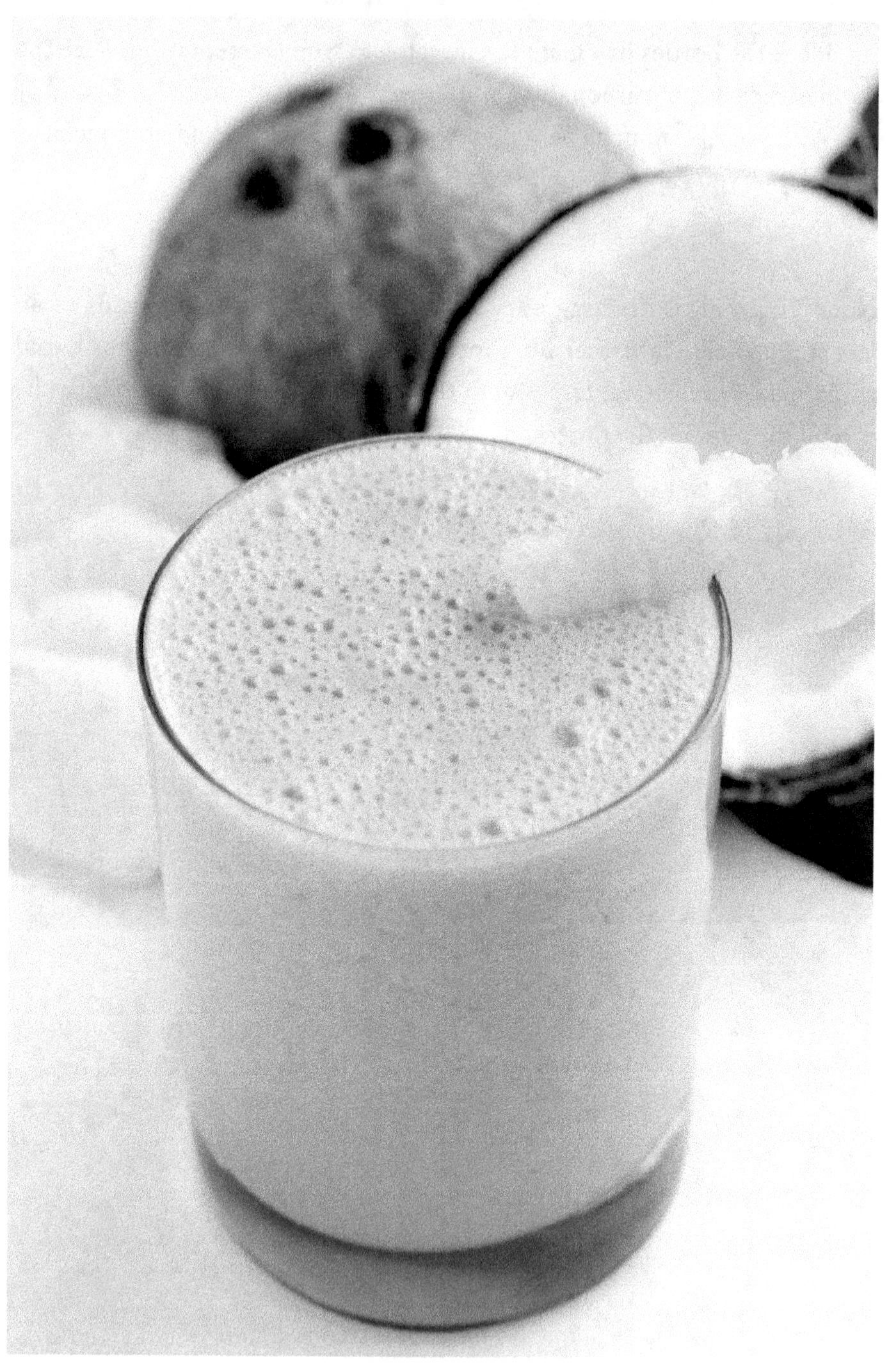

Ingredients:

- 1 cup fresh or frozen pineapple chunks
- 1/2 cup coconut milk (canned for creaminess)
- 1/2 cup fresh spinach leaves
- 1/2 banana (optional, for added sweetness and creaminess)
- 1/2 cup plain Greek yogurt1 tablespoon chia seeds (optional, for added texture and nutrition)
- Ice cubes (optional)

Instructions:

1. If you are using newly peeled pineapple, then peel it and cut it into pieces. When using frozen pineapple, nothing needs to be done.

2. Then in a blender add pineapple chunks, coconut milk, a handful of fresh spinach leaves, a banana if using, Greek yogurt and chia seeds.

3. Mix all the ingredients until the mixture is homogeneous. After that, if you desire a colder and thicker smoothie, add ice cubes.

3. It should apparently taste somewhat sourish and in order to either adjust it according to its sweetness or thickness by adding more pineapple, banana or coconut milk.

4. Smoothie for green pineapple coconut, pour into the glass.

5. However, add more of these chunks in pineapple, shredded coconut and sprinkle of chia seeds at the chaidetails for a touch of adornment.

6. Feast at the amazingly nutritional value contained in the Green Pineapple Coconut Smoothie as you sip and enjoy it.

Super easy? To suit your needs, you may customize this smoothie by changing ingredient portions. It is an attractive combination of ripe pineapple and coconut, sweet and creamy that also provides essential green elements. Of course, it fits perfectly as a fast and healthy breakfast, or a delightful snack.

5.4.4 Apple, Carrot and Celery Smoothie

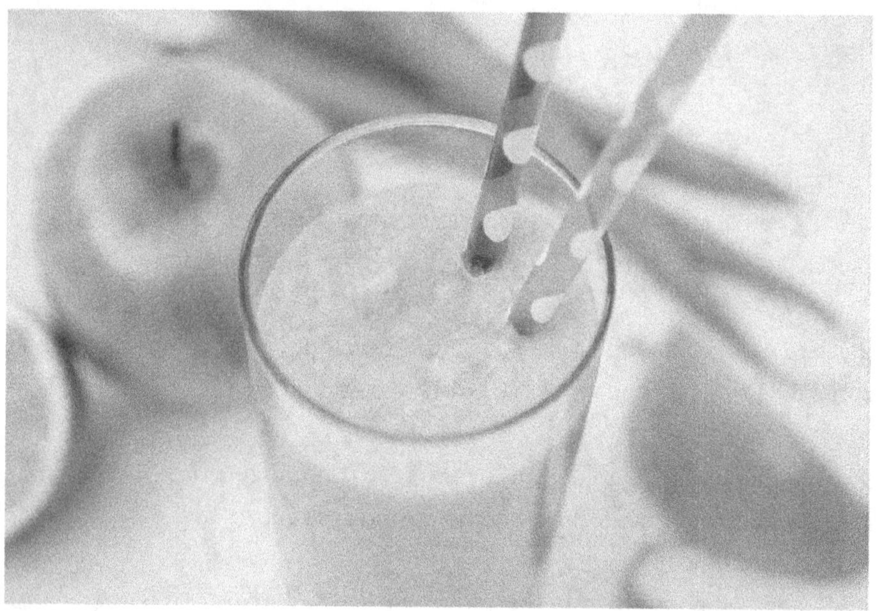

Ingredients:

- 2 apples, cored and diced (leave the skin for added fiber)
- 2 carrots, peeled and grated
- 2 celery stalks, finely chopped
- 1/4 cup raisins or dried cranberries (optional, for sweetness)
- 1/4 cup chopped walnuts or almonds (optional, for crunch)
- Juice of 1 lemon
- 2 tablespoons
- Greek yogurt or mayonnaise (adjust to your preference)
- 1 tablespoon honey or maple syrup (optional, for added sweetness)
- Salt and pepper to taste

Instructions:

1. Prepare Ingredients:

Cut the apples into dice, peel and finely chop the carrots, then dice the celery finely.

2. Combine Ingredients: Place the diced apples, chopped almonds, raisins or dried cranberries, shredded carrots, and chopped celery in a big bowl.

3. Get the dressing ready: Whisk together the lemon juice, mayonnaise or Greek yogurt, honey (if using), salt, and pepper in a small bowl.

4. Combine Dressing and Salad: Drizzle the dressing over the blend of apples, carrots, and celery.

5. Mix Gently: Gently mix the ingredients together until the dressing coats everything.

6. Chill (Optional): Before serving, the salad can be chilled for about 30 minutes to bring out the flavors.

7. Serve: Transfer the apple-carrot-celery salad into dishes or plates using a spoon.

8. Savor: As a light and healthful snack or side dish, savor this crisp and refreshing salad!

5.4.5 Berry Banana Spinach Smoothie

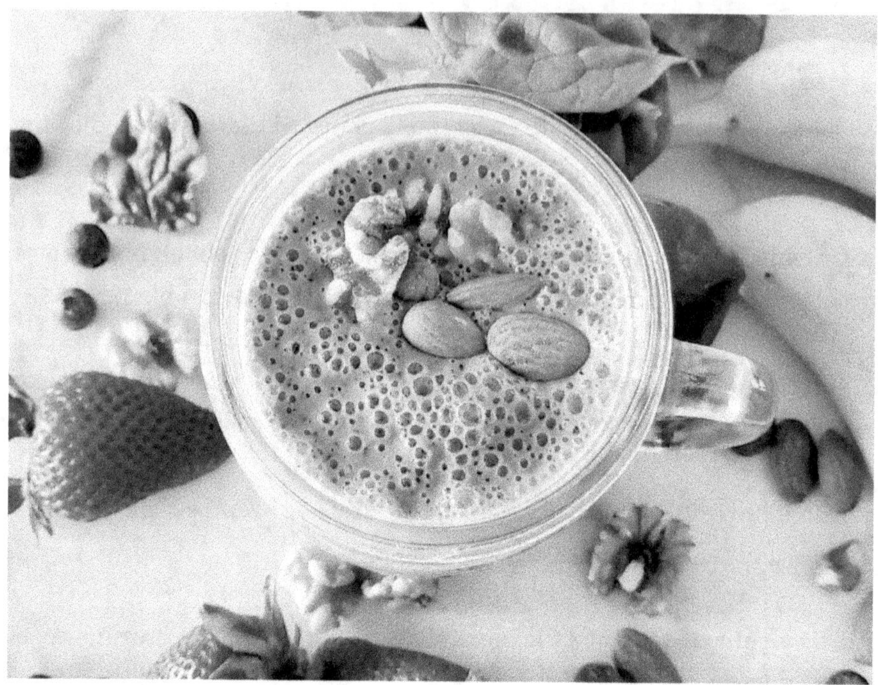

Ingredients:

- 1 cup fresh or frozen mixed berries (strawberries, blueberries, raspberries)
- 1 ripe banana
- 1 cup fresh spinach leaves
- 1/2 cup Greek yogurt (plain or vanilla)
- 1/2 cup almond milk (or any milk of your choice)
- 1 tablespoon chia seeds (optional, for added texture and nutrition)
- Ice cubes (optional)

Instructions:

1. Prepare Ingredients: If you use fresh berries, they should be washed. If the banana has already ripened we must cut and eliminate its peel.

2. Blend: Pile the mixed berries, banana chunks, ice cubes, Greek yogurt,

almond milk, fresh spinach leaves and (if have) chia seeds into a blender.

3. Blend Until Smooth: Blend all the ingredients in a blender until you get a creamy smooth texture.

4. Taste and alter: On your desired, make the smoothie thicker or sweeter, depending on your preferences. If required, add some more honey or more pieces of banana.

5. Serve: Pour the Berry Banana Spinach Smoothie into a glass.

6. Optional Garnish: Choice of appearance is topping with a chia seeds sprinkling or a few whole berries.

7. Enjoy: Drink this vibrant, nutrient boosting smoothie.

Not only does it combine the zest of berries, the gentleness of bananas, and the health benefits of spinach. It provides you pleasure when used as a hot snack or when you want a refreshing beginning of the day. You are free to change the recipe to suit you by adjusting the choice of fruit, nut butter, or protein powder.

5.5 Dessert Recipes

5.5.1 Low-carb Chocolate Mousse

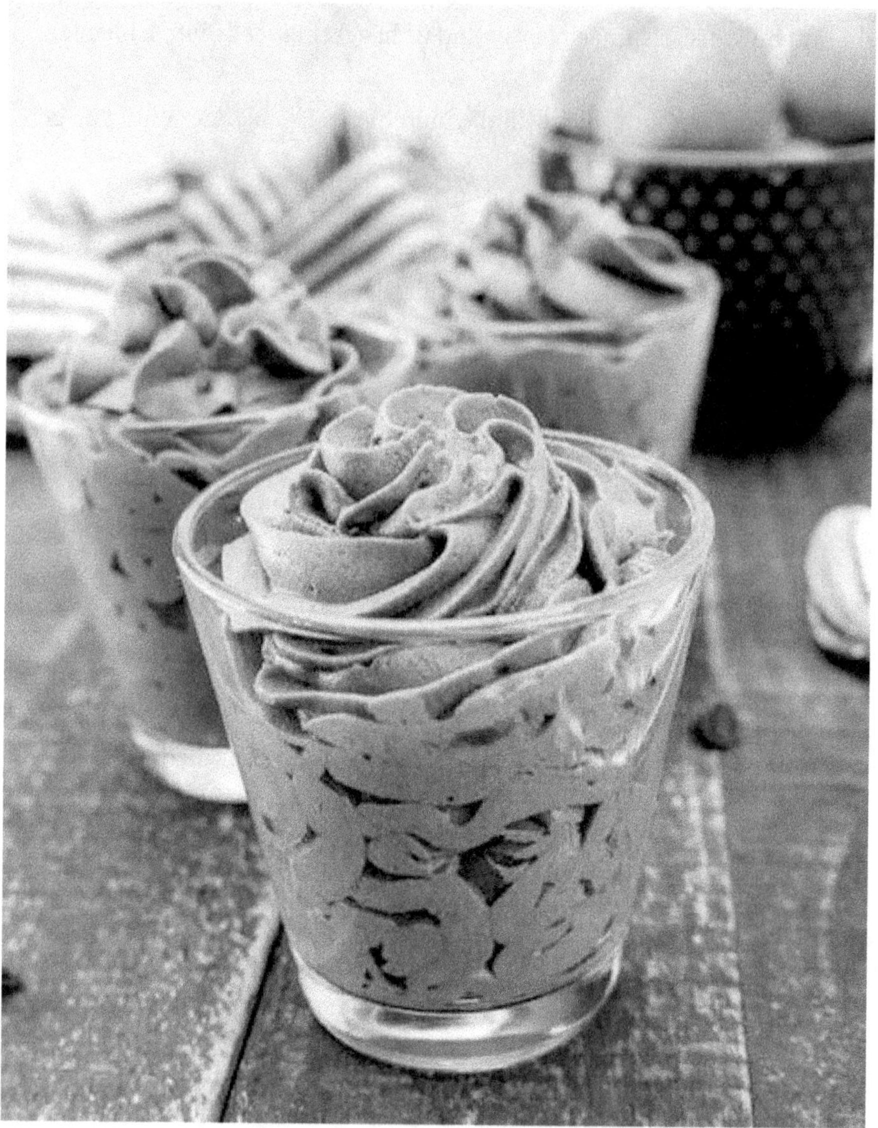

Ingredients:

- One cup thick cream
- 1/4 cup chocolate powder, unsweetened
- 1/4 cup of your preferred low-carb sweetener, or powdered erythritol
- 1 teaspoon of vanilla extract

- A dash of salt
- Shavings of dark chocolate or shredded chocolate (optional garnish)

Instructions:

1. Chill a mixing bowl, beaters, or whisk attachment in the fridge for a minimum of fifteen minutes.

2. Beat the heavy cream until firm peaks form in the cooled basin. Take care not to whisk the cream too much; stop whipping when it becomes thick and stiff.

3. Sift or whisk the unsweetened cocoa powder, vanilla extract, powdered erythritol, and a little amount of salt together in a another dish until thoroughly mixed.

4. Gently fold in the chocolate mixture until thoroughly combined. To preserve the light and airy texture of the mousse, fold with a spatula.

5. To help the chocolate mousse firm and take on flavor, cover the bowl and place it in the refrigerator for at least two hours.

6. Spoon the low-carb chocolate mousse into bowls or glasses for serving when it has chilled.

7. You may top with grated chocolate or dark chocolate shavings, if you'd like.

8. Treat yourself to this rich and creamy low-carb chocolate mousse for a filling dessert.

This recipe is perfect for anyone on a low-carb or ketogenic diet since it makes a delicious chocolate dessert with little carbohydrates. Change the amount of sweetener used to get the sweetness you like. Have fun!

5.5.2 Healthy Blackberry Cobbler

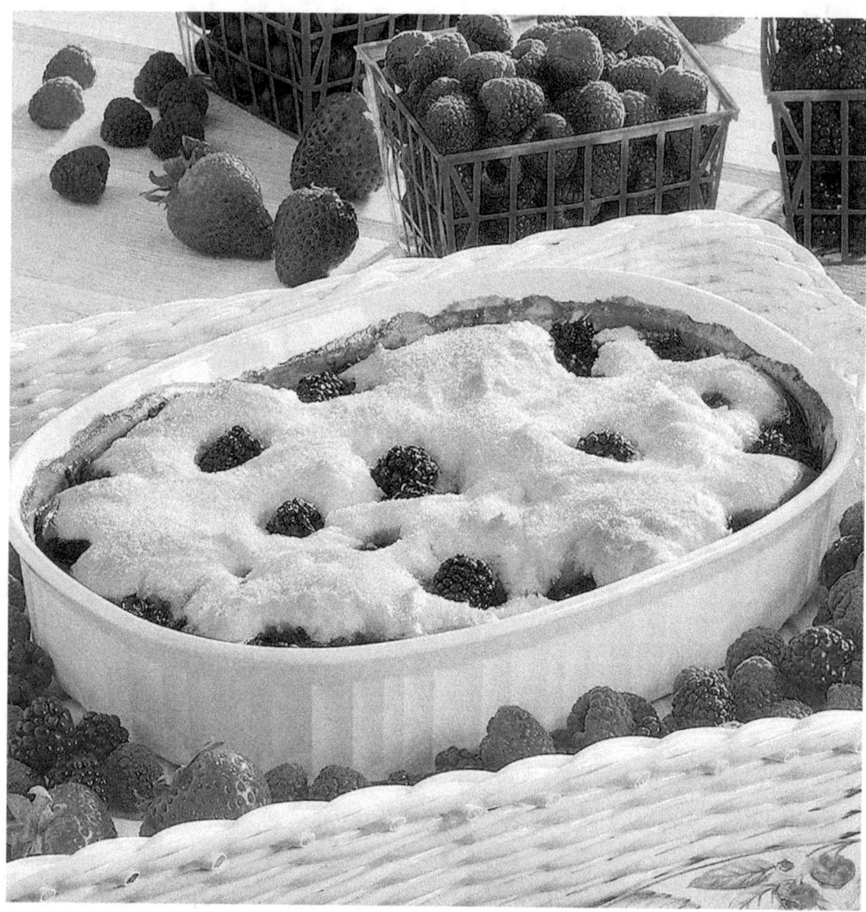

Ingredients:

- For the Filling
- 4 cups fresh blackberries
- ¼ cup honey or maple syrup
- 1 teaspoon vanilla extract

- 2 teaspoons cornstarch or arrowroot powder
- The zing of 1 lemon

- For the Topping:
- 1 cup of moment oats
- 1/4 cup almond flour
- 1/2 cup entire wheat flour
- 1/4 cup coconut oil that has liquefied
- 1/4 cup honey or maple syrup
- 1 teaspoon of baking powder
- ½ teaspoon ground cinnamon
- Pinch of salt

Instructions:

1. Preheat Oven: Turn the oven's temperature up to 350°F/175°C.

2. In an enormous bowl, cautiously mix together honey, maple syrup, arrowroot powder, cornstarch, vanilla substance, and lemon zing until the blackberries are totally covered.

3. Move the blackberry blend to a baking dish and smooth it out equally.

4. In a different dish, combine as one the oats, almond flour, entire wheat flour, honey, maple syrup, softened coconut oil, baking powder, cinnamon, and a little spot of salt. Consolidate the fixings and mix until brittle.

5. Add Topping to Berries: Over the blackberry filling, evenly distribute the oat topping.

6. Bake in a preheated oven for 30 to 35 minutes, or until the garnish is

brilliant brown and the blackberry filling is percolating.

7. Permit the cobbler to cool for a couple of moments prior to serving.

8. Serve the healthy blackberry cobbler warm, maybe with a scoop of Greek yogurt or a touch of whipped cream on top.

Improved with honey or maple syrup, this nutritious blackberry shoemaker uses a lot of fiber from the oats and entire wheat flour. Partake in a wonton pastry faultless!

5.5.3 Avocado Chocolate Truffles

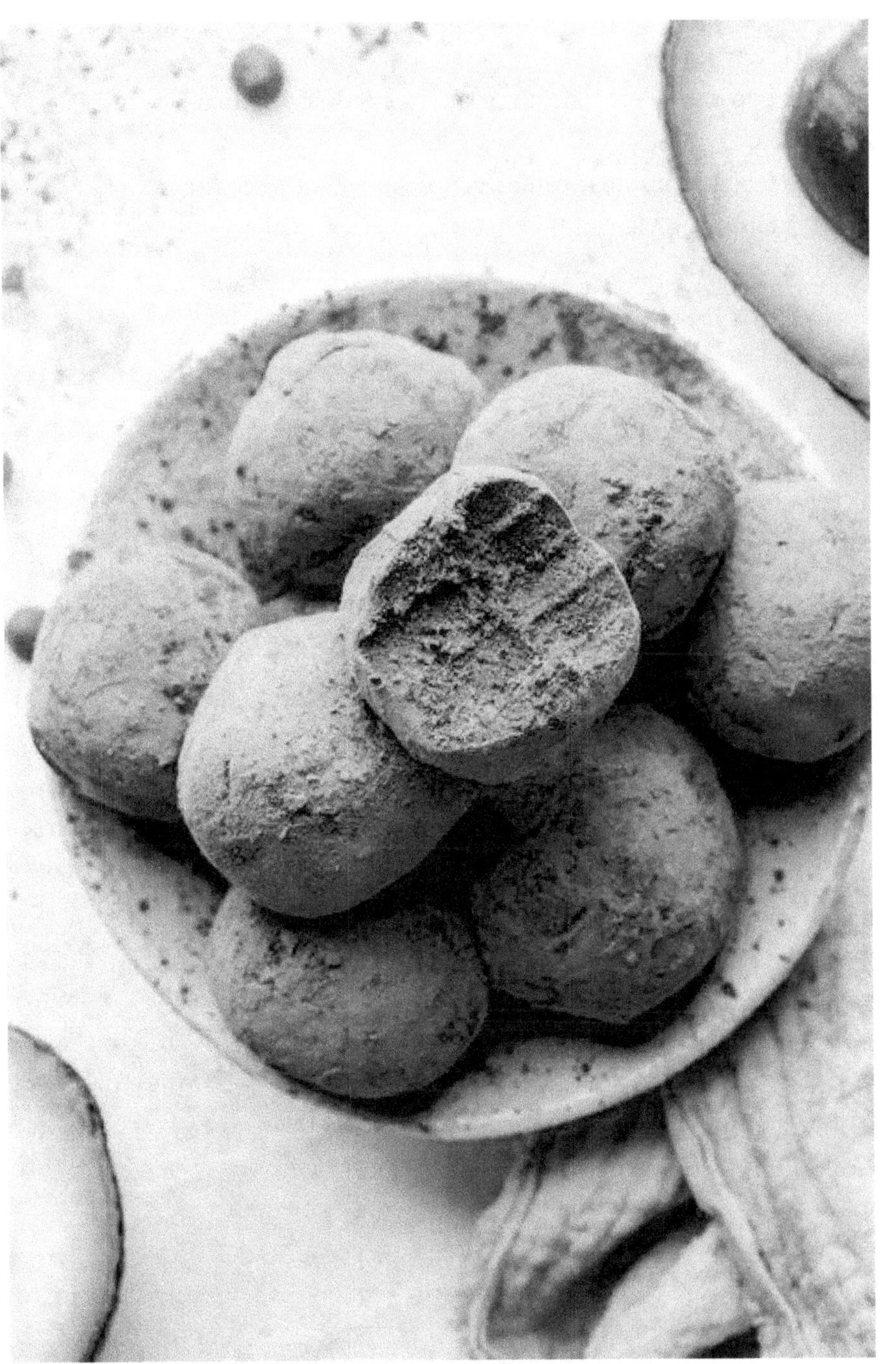

Ingredients:

- 2 ripe avocados
- 1/2 cup dark chocolate chips or chopped dark chocolate (at least 70% cocoa)
- 2-3 tablespoons unsweetened cocoa powder (for coating)
- 1-2 tablespoons maple syrup or agave nectar (adjust to taste)
- 1 teaspoon vanilla extract
- A pinch of salt

Instructions:

1. Melt dark chocolate chips stirring occasionally in a double boiler, or until smooth in a microwave in short bursts. Let it cool down slightly.

2. Mash well-ripened avocados in a separate bowl until they reach a smooth consistency. Also, for consistency, use a blender or fork.

3. Combine the mashed avocados with the melted chocolate, vanilla extract, maple syrup or agave nectar, and a pinch of salt. When all components have been appropriately incorporated, mix thoroughly.

4. Keep the mixture refrigerated for thirty to sixty minutes, until it solidifies.

5. Once the mix hardens, cut is into small chunks and roll into the size of truffle balls for consumption in a single bite. Set them on a paper-lined tray.

6. Round each truffle with unsweetened cocoa powder.

7. The truffles are allowed to soften a little when shaping, keep them in the fridge for a while to solidify.

8. Set the avocado chocolate truffles on a tray and indulge on a creamy and

dreamy treat!

5.5.4 Frozen Banana Ice cream

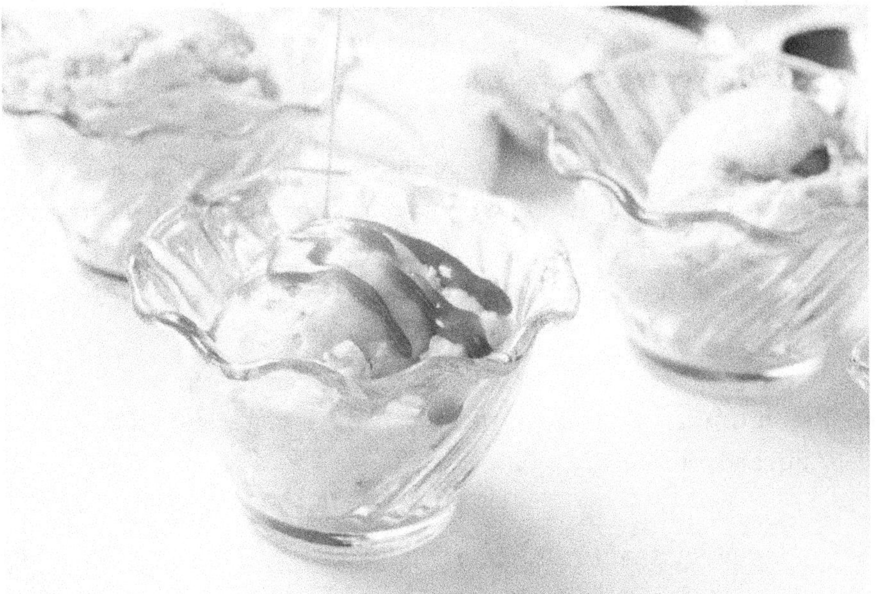

Ingredients:

- 4 ripe bananas, peeled and sliced into coins
- 1 teaspoon vanilla extract (optional)
- Toppings of your choice (such as nuts, berries, chocolate chips, or honey, optional)

Instructions:

1. Peal the ripe bananas and cut them into coins. Ensure the banana cuts are not contacting as you organize them on a plate or dish covered with

paper. Freeze until strong, or for like two hours.

2. Put the frozen banana cuts into a strong food processor or blender. On the off chance that utilizing, add the vanilla concentrate.

3. Process the frozen banana cuts in a blender until they are velvety and smooth. Intermittently, you could have to delay and scratch down the sides. It will ultimately transform into a rich consistency likened to delicately served frozen yogurt, so show restraint.

4. Go ahead and top with chocolate chips, berries, almonds, or a honey sprinkle in the event that you'd like. Pulse the blender briefly to incorporate.

5. Immediately serve the banana frozen yogurt by scooping it into dishes or cones.

6. Relish this irreproachable frozen banana frozen yogurt that is both delicious and refreshing.

5.5.5 Honey Roasted Fruit Salad

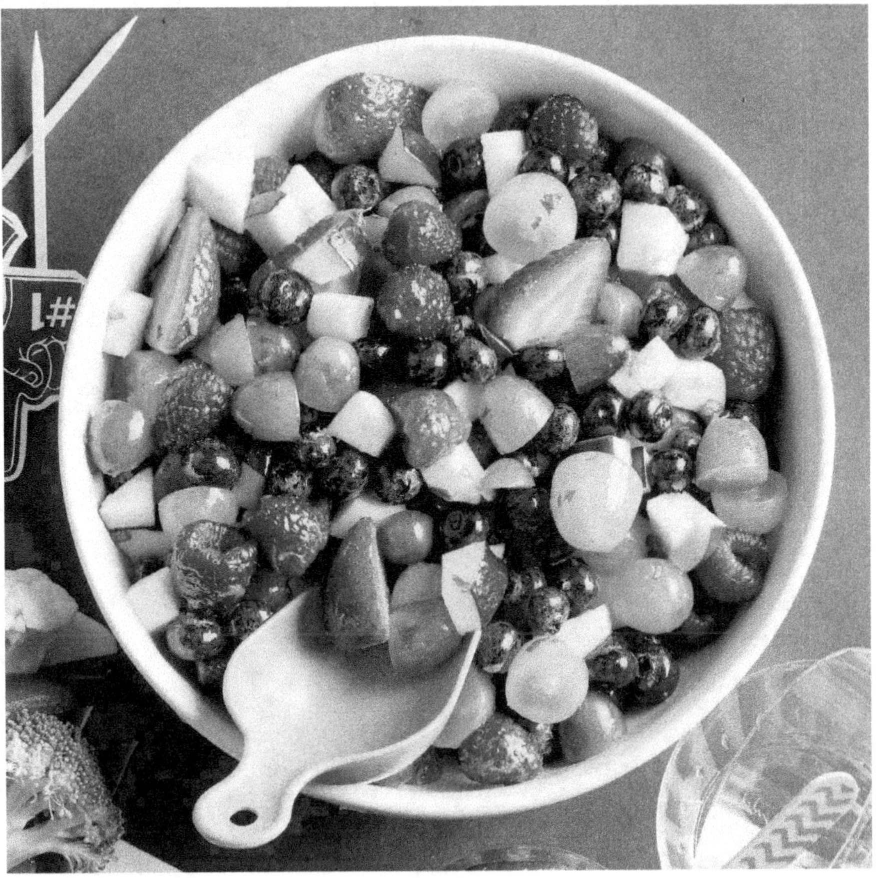

Ingredients:

- For the Roasted Fruit:
- 2 cups mixed fresh fruits (such as strawberries, pineapple chunks, grapes, and kiwi)
- 2 tablespoons honey
- 1 tablespoon melted coconut oil or olive oil
- 1 teaspoon vanilla extract

- For the Salad:

- 2 cups mixed salad greens (arugula, spinach, or your choice)
- 1/4 cup crumbled feta cheese or goat cheese
- 1/4 cup chopped nuts (walnuts, almonds, or pecans)
- Fresh mint leaves for garnish (optional)

- For the Dressing:
- 2 tablespoons balsamic vinegar
- 1 tablespoon honey
- 2 tablespoons extra virgin olive oil
- Salt and pepper to taste

Instructions:

1. Preheat oven. Set the oven's temperature to 400°F, or 200°C.

2. Blend the fresh fruits combination, honey, vanilla embodiment, and warmed coconut or olive oil in a bowl. Toss the fruits until they are evenly coated.

3. Arrange the covered natural products on a material paper-lined baking sheet. Roast the fruits for 15 to 20 minutes, or until they are caramelized and starting to become brown, in a preheated stove. For even roasting, stir every once in a while.

4. In a little bowl, combine one balsamic vinegar, honey, additional virgin olive oil, salt, and pepper to make the dressing while the fruits are roasting. Set aside.

5. Arrange the blended plate of mixed salad greens in a major bowl. Put the simmered fruits on top.

6. Top the plate of mixed salad greens with cleaved nuts and disintegrated feta or goat cheese.

7. Drizzle the prepared balsamic honey dressing over the salad.

8. You might add new mint leaves as an enhancement on the off chance that you'd like. Tenderly prepare the serving of mixed salad greens to consolidate the flavors in general.

9. Enjoy the mouthwatering contrast of fresh salad greens, honey-roasted fruits, and a rich dressing as soon as possible.

6

Chapter 6

Beyond the 21 Days

6.1 Long-term Approaches to Intermittent Fasting

The way to long-term intermittent fasting is to coordinate fasting cycles into your everyday schedule consistently. For a IF routine that is feasible, remember the accompanying focuses:

1. Select a Period for Maintainable Fasting: Pick a window for fasting in light of your preferences and lifestyle. The 16/8 strategy (16 hours of fasting, 8 hours of eating) and the 5:2 technique (comprising of five days of customary eating followed by two days of calorie limitation) are two well known approaches.

2. Pay attention to Your Body: Focus on the prompts that come from your body. In the event that a particular fasting procedure appears to be excessively confining or awkward, ponder changing your system. Finding an equilibrium that suits you is fundamental.

3. Remain Hydrated: During times of fasting, drink a lot of water to stay

hydrated. Dark espresso and natural teas are habitually allowed and can be utilized to control craving.

4. Make meals high in nutrients a priority: During eating times, focus on nutrient-dense meals to ensure that you meet your nutritional needs. An even eating routine ought to contain a scope of organic products, vegetables, lean meats, and whole grains.

5. Utilize Physical Activity: Make customary activity a piece of your everyday timetable. Because it helps control weight and improves general health, intermittent fasting can be used in conjunction with exercise.

6. Slow Implementation: Consider starting slowly if you have never done intermittent fasting before. Start with shorter fasting windows and gradually increase them as your body gets used to them.

7. Consistency is Key: Consistency is essential to long-term success. Keep up with the irregular fasting plan you have laid out, yet allow yourself to wander as the need might arise. Changes in your timetable or extraordinary occasions can be obliged with changes.

8. Check on Progress: Record any progressions in weight, energy level, or general prosperity, as well as any profound changes. This could help you in deciding how effective your picked intermittent fasting system is.

9. Seek the advice of a medical professional: It's ideal to talk with a certified dietitian or other medical services supplier prior to making any huge dietary changes, especially in the event that you have any fundamental clinical diseases or concerns.

10. Join with a Decent Lifestyle: The best outcomes from irregular fasting come from a sound, balanced way of life. Ensure you get sufficient rest, figure out how to deal with pressure, and keep a hopeful attitude toward

your overall well-being.

11. Notice the Planning of Nutrients: At the point when you consume supplements inside your eating window, focus on the planning of it. To ensure a reliable stock of supplements over the course of the day, split your dinners and tidbits.

12. Include all-natural foods: Place serious areas of strength for an in your eating routine on entire, negligibly handled food varieties. To advance general wellbeing, incorporate a scope of lively leafy foods, entire grains, lean meats, and solid fats.

13. Plan Dinners in Ahead: Improving food choices and keeping away from rash decisions during your eating window might be accomplished by arranging your dinners ahead of time. Set up your feasts ahead of time for more straightforwardness.

14. Attempt Different Approaches: There are a few ways to deal with irregular fasting. Evaluate numerous methodologies to see which best suits your preferences and lifestyle. Some people may succeed by fasting every day, while others may prefer to fast on alternate days.

15. Oversee Stress: Delayed pressure can unfavorably affect your overall wellbeing and may make it more hard for you to keep a intermittent fasting plan. Incorporate pressure decrease systems into your regular daily schedule, like yoga, profound breathing, or reflection.

16. Recognize Small Victories: Recognize and celebrate the non-scale triumphs, such higher state of mind, better mental lucidity, and more energy. It's possible that these beneficial changes will have the same effect as weight changes.

17. Ordinary Wellbeing Check-ups: Make an arrangement for routine

clinical assessments to watch out for your general prosperity. In the event that you are making significant dietary or way of life changes, or on the other hand assuming you have any previous clinical issues, this is particularly urgent.

18. Teach Yourself: Keep on finding out about the basics of nourishment, prosperity, and intermittent fasting. Knowing the science hidden irregular fasting will engage you to settle on wellbeing related choices with information.

19. Change based on life stages: Comprehend that things could change throughout everyday life, and you might have to adjust your intermittent fasting technique accordingly. Be versatile and alter your timetable to oblige different phases of life.

20. Establish a Support Group: Long haul achievement could profit from having an encouraging group of people. Discuss your targets with friends and family, or contemplate joining on the web bunches where you might associate with others who are fast and irregular.

Remember that not every person can profit from Intermittent fasting, and that everybody's response is unique. For long-term adherence and achievement, it's basic to distinguish a system that supplements your preferences, general way of life, and well-being objectives.

6.2 Looking Forward to a Healthier You

1. Journaling about Gratitude: Write down your appreciation in a diary. List the benefits of your IF journey that you are grateful for in terms of your life and health. Expressing appreciation might improve your general feeling of wellbeing.

2. Plan an Adventure: Arrange a trip or adventure that focuses on fitness.

Pick an activity that fits with your renewed energy and endurance, whether it's a yoga retreat, a weekend cycle excursion, or a hike.

3. Practice Mindful Meditation: Use meditation to bring mindfulness into your celebration. To stay in the present while appreciating the path you've traveled and the improvements you've seen, practice mindfulness meditation.

4. Host a Virtual party: If socializing in person is difficult for you, organize a virtual party for your loved ones. Using video conversations or online resources, rejoice with each other and share your experiences and journey.

5. Make a Customized Award or Certificate: Create a diploma or trophy that represents your accomplishments with your own design. It can be a funny diploma for being a "Master of Fasting" or a prize for being a "Commitment to Health" recipient. Show it out with pride as a physical memento of your accomplishment.

6. Attend a Fitness Class or Workshop: Take part in an exercise class or workshop that deviates from your customary schedule. Attending a dancing class or martial arts workshop, for example, might be a novel way to commemorate your fitness journey.

7. Artistic Expression: Use art to communicate your trip. Make a piece of art—a painting, a sculpture, or anything else—that captures your metamorphosis and the benefits of sporadic fasting.

8. Create a Health Manifesto: Write out your beliefs and aspirations for your well-being in a manifesto. To help you keep focused on your health goals, use this as a guide and refer to it often.

9. Symbolic Release Ceremony: Plan a symbolic release ceremony to let go of any bad habits or ideas that have impeded your efforts to improve your health. This might entail putting challenges in writing and burning or

dumping them ceremoniously.

10. Dance Is A Great Way To Express Yourself: Have a dance party to celebrate! Create a playlist with your top upbeat songs and dance your way through your accomplishments. Dancing is a fantastic kind of exercise as well as a happy expression.

11. Make Your Own Exercise Playlist: Create a playlist specifically for your workouts that represents your journey. Add upbeat and motivational tunes to create a soundtrack that reflects the good changes in your life.

12. Organize a Day of Retreat: Set aside a day for introspection and rest. Take time to enjoy yourself, detach from everyday worries, and recognize the strides you've made on your IF journey.

13. Share Your Knowledge: Use this chance to impart what you've learned about intermittent fasting. Whether it's via a blog, social media, or conversations with friends, sharing your experiences may make a meaningful difference.

Honoring your IF journey means appreciating the work you've put into your health and welcoming the beneficial developments that have occurred. Make your celebration memorable and pleasurable by designing it to suit your tastes and personality.

Conclusion

As you wind up this program, I invite you to take a minute to visualize your life as a painting, where each brushstroke reflects your health, awareness, and harmony. Just like how a painter meticulously picks each color to build a masterpiece, you too can construct a beautiful life by accepting the obstacles as chances for growth and celebrating in your achievements, no matter how apparently little they may be. Remember, your path towards wellness is an adventure that lasts a lifetime, and this 21-day plan is just the beginning of it.

As you move forward, I hope the basic ideals that you have fostered during this program become an important part of your life. The quest of health, moments of self-kindness, and self-discovery are all vital elements for a healthy and happy existence. Cherish the equilibrium that you have established and allow it to pervade every part of your life. May the decisions you make bring you strength, and may the everyday habits that nurture your mind, body, and soul offer you joy.

Throughout this guide, you have learnt vital lessons and built resilience. Take these with you as you begin on the next part of your path towards wellness. Your road towards wellness is a constant tale of personal improvement and happiness. My goal for you is that every thread of your life is braided with a feeling of purpose, meaningful connections, and wonderful health. May you continue to inspire everyone around you and leave behind a legacy of vigor.

As the chapters of "Wellness Beyond 40" come to a close, I want to remind you that the tale of your well-being continues unwritten. Every day gives a fresh chance to cultivate a healthier, more vibrant self. Remember, the path towards wellness is not a destination, but a constant practice of self-improvement. May you continue to welcome this experience with open arms, and may the following years of your life be filled with robust health, boundless joy, and a legacy of well-lived years.

P.S: Please do not forget to leave your comments on Amazon as you have read this book. I would love to read all your feedbacks.